# What People Are Saying About
# *Karma Chow*

"Every recipe in this book is the kind I want to feed myself and my family over and over again. Wholesome, creative, delicious, easy, and will lead me to bliss."

—**Christy Morgan,** "The Blissful Chef,"
author of *Blissful Bites: Vegan Meals That
Nourish Mind, Body, and Planet*

"Melissa's orientation towards healthy vegan cooking is user friendly and fun. I highly recommend this delicious and accessible cookbook. *Karma Chow* makes cooking a joy!"

—**Mandy Ingber**,
celebrity yoga teacher and
creator of Yogalosophy

"Melissa Costello brings joy to cooking. The cookbook radiates with happy, healthy, and vibrant dishes that are a clear indication of her love of life and fabulous, healthful food. This is the cookbook for anyone looking to get on a path to wellness without sacrificing flavor and fun!"

—**Carolyn Scott-Hamilton**, holistic nutritionist,
plant-based chef, author of *The Healthy Voyager's
Global Kitchen Cookbook*, speaker and creator/host
of The Healthy Voyager shows, site, and brand

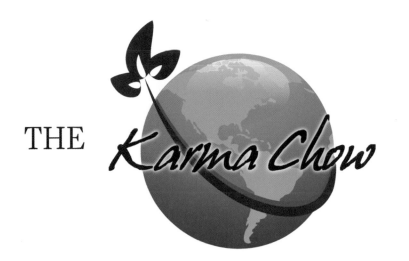

# THE Karma Chow

# ULTIMATE COOKBOOK

125+ Plant-Based Vegan Recipes for a Fit, Happy, Healthy You

MELISSA COSTELLO
founder, KarmaChow.com

**Health Communications, Inc.**
**Deerfield Beach, Florida**

*www.hcibooks.com*

**Library of Congress Cataloging-in-Publication Data
is available from the Library of Congress.**

ISBN-13: 978-0-7573-1633-3 (paperback)
ISBN-10: 0-7573-1633-6 (paperback)
ISBN-13: 978-0-7573-1634-0 (e-book)
ISBN-10: 0-7573-1634-4 (e-book)

Publisher: Health Communications, Inc.
3201 S.W. 15th Street
Deerfield Beach, FL 33442–8190

*Photography by Kelsey Skiver © kelseymariephoto.com*
*Cover design by Larissa Hise Henoch*
*Interior design and formatting by Lawna Patterson Oldfield*

# Contents

Foreword by Tony Horton, Creator of P90X® • xi

Introduction: The Journey to Plant-Based Eating,
   Optimal Health, and Vivacious Vitality • 1
   ◆ *My Journey to Plant-Based Eating* ◆ *My Food Philosophy*
   ◆ *The Great Food Disconnect* ◆ *Kitchen & Pantry Essentials*
   ◆ *Healthy Pantry Must-Haves* ◆ *Beans: Buying in Bulk or in a Can?*
   ◆ *Spices & Herbs* ◆ *Unusual yet Useful Staples*
   ◆ *What About Baking?* ◆ *Find Your Fun in the Kitchen*

Chapter 1: *Plant-Based Breakfasts and Beverages*
Quinoa Protein Brekkie Bowl • 25
Apricot Tea Muffins • 27
Banana Chocolate Chip Minis • 29
Veggie Breakfast Scramble • 31
Karmic Cherry Almond Granola • 33
Tempeh Sausage Patties • 35
Buckwheat Corn Cakes with Blueberry Drizzle • 37
   *Blueberry Drizzle* • 37
Rise and Shine Granola Parfaits • 39
Cold Cinnamon Oaty Cereal • 40
Cashew Milk • 41

Banana Chia Pancakes with Coconut Crème Sauce • 43

   *Coconut Crème Sauce* • 43

Da Bomb Fruity Smoothie • 44

Healer Ginger Tea • 45

Minty Hot Chocolate • 45

Cherry Chocolate Smoothie • 47

Green Heaven Smoothie • 49

Divine Coconutty Chai (Caffeine Free) • 51

Cherry Pecan Quinoa Muffins • 53

Pumpkin Pie Waffles • 55

Gluten-Free Zucchini Bread • 56

## Chapter 2: *Nosh, Nibble, and Dip Away*

Thai-Style Tempeh Lettuce Wraps • 59

Stuffed Mushroom Poppers • 61

Veggie Seed Roll-Ups • 63

Kickin' Edamame Dip • 65

Garnet Hummus • 67

Green Earth Dip • 69

Heart-Full Bruschetta • 71

Artichoke and White Bean Dip with Rosemary • 73

Arriba Black Bean Dip • 75

Sunflower Seed "Pâté" • 77

Spicy Olive Tapenade • 78

Cheezy Popcorn • 79

Creamy Spinach Artichoke Dip • 81

Roasted and Spiced Mixed Nuts • 83

Peanut Sauce • 84

Chipotle Cashew Cheeze Sauce • 85

Sweet and Savory Kale "Chips" • 86

Charlie's Tomato Sauce Marinara · 87

Savory Golden Mushroom Gravy · 88

Chile Ranchero Sauce · 89

Dreamy Avocado "Mayo" · 90

## Chapter 3: *Hearty One-Pot Soups and Stews*

Lentil Soup · 93

Indian-Spiced Coconut Yam Soup · 95

"Feeling Tropical" Black Bean Soup · 96

Kitchen Sink Veggie Soup · 97

Holy Moly Green Gazpacho · 99

Chowdery Corn Soup · 101

Golden Split Pea Soup · 102

Cream of Celery Soup · 103

Dreamy Roasted Butternut Squash Soup · 104

Curried Veggie "Stoup" · 106

Kinda Like Mom's Beefy Stew · 107

Garlicky White Bean and Kale Soup · 109

Dill-icious Roasted Carrot Cauliflower Soup · 111

Smoky Tempeh Chili · 112

## Chapter 4: *Succulent Salads and Delicious Dressings*

Brussels Sprouts Salad · 115

*Lemon Vinaigrette* · 115

Raw Kale Salad with Creamy Chipotle Dressing · 117

*Creamy Chipotle Dressing* · 117

Quinoa Tabbouleh · 119

Wild Rice Salad with Balsamic Maple Dressing · 121

*Balsamic Maple Dressing* · 121

Dilled Potato Salad · 122

Herb-Infused Chickpea Salad • 123

   *Herbed Lemon Dressing* • 123

Quinoa and Strawberry Salad with Lime Vinaigrette • 125

   *Lime Vinaigrette* • 125

Raw Thai Slaw ◆ *Thai Dressing* • 127

Kale Slaw with Creamy Pumpkin Seed Dressing • 129

   *Creamy Pumpkin Seed Dressing* • 129

Spinach Salad with "Bacon" and Creamy

   Tahini Dressing ◆ *Creamy Tahini Dressing* • 131

White Bean Zucchini Salad • 132

Mixed Baby Greens with Walnut, Pear,

   and Pomegranate Mint Dressing • 133

   *Pomegranate Mint Dressing* • 133

Vegan Caesar Salad ◆ *Caesar Dressing* ◆ *Vegan Parmesan* • 134

## Chapter 5: *Main Dish Favorites: Veganized*

Pasta and "Meat"balls • 137

Korean-Style Tempeh Tacos with Coleslaw • 139

   *Coleslaw* ◆ *Dijon Dressing* • 139

Soba Noodle Stir-Fry in Creamy Cashew Sauce • 141

   *Cashew Sauce* • 141

Un-Shepherd's Pie • 143

   *Mashed Topping* • 142

   *Tempeh Veggie Filling* • 143

Pad Thai in Peanut Coconut Sauce • 144

   *Peanut Coconut Sauce* • 144

Greek Tomato Burgers • 145

Mac and Ch-ch-cheeeeze • 147

Lemon Dill Aioli Dipping Sauce • 148

Chickpea Fillets • 149

Veggie Loaf with Tomato Glaze • 150

Baja-Style Fajitas • 153

Baked Ziti with Spinach • 154

Cashew Ricotta Cheeze • 154

Suprem-oh Burrito • 155

Chickpea "Tuna" Salad • 157

Curried Tempeh Salad • 158

Fresh Pesto, Tomato, and Zucchini Pasta  *Cilantro Pesto*  159

Quinoa and Currant Stuffed Bell Peppers • 161

Karma Burgers with Chipotle Mayo • 163

   *Chipotle Mayo* • 163

Cha-Cha Enchiladarole • 164

## Chapter 6: *Simply Sublime Sides*

Wild Mushroom Quinoa Pilaf • 169

Cranberry Balsamic Green Beans • 171

Norwegian Sweet and Sour Cabbage • 172

Apple Cherry Chutney • 173

Soba Noodle and Pea Pesto • 175

Maple Miso Brussels Sprouts • 177

Chili Sweet Potato Batons • 178

Spaghetti Squash Italiano • 179

Creamy Tahini Kale • 181

   *Tahini Sauce* • 181

Mashed Coconut Yams with Cardamom • 183

Blissed-Out Herb-Roasted Taters • 185

Cilantro Cauliflower Smash • 186

Hurried Curried Greens • 187

Spicy Garlic Spinach • 189

Cumin Cauliflower Roast • 191

## Chapter 7: *Ooey, Gooey, and Delightfully Decadent Desserts*

Black Bean Brownie Bites • 195

Choco Chocolate Chip Avo Pudding • 197

Euphoria Nuggets • 199

Strawberry Crème Mousse with Pistachio Topping • 201
   *Pistachio Topping* • 201

Almond Berry Crème Parfaits • 203
   *Raw Almond Frangipane Crème* • 203
   *Raspberry Sauce* • 203

Decadent Banana Carob Bread Pudding • 204
   *Cashew/Almond Milk* • 205

Coconut Anise Almond Cookies • 207
   *Chocolate Topping* • 207

Apple/Pear Crisp • 209
   *Crumb Topping* • 208

Cardamom-Scented Chocolate Chippers • 211

Divine Chocolate Truffles • 212

Peanut Butter Cookies • 213

Chocolaty Rice Krispy Thingies • 215

Luscious Limey "Cheese"cake • 217
   *Crust* ◆ *Filling* • 217

Lavender Coconut Ice Cream • 219

Coconut Whipped Cream • 220

Vanilla Scented Balsamic Figs • 221

Baked Coconut Ginger Millet Pudding • 222


Baking Substitutions 101 • 223

Resources and Recommendations • 227

Books and Films • 231

Acknowledgments • 233

About the Author • 235

Index • 237

# Foreword

*A* *hhhh, food! I love it.* It makes me happy! But I'm not just an
enthusiastic eater; I'm also a smart eater. And if you're reading
this now, so are you (or you're about to be).

I'm a fitness guy, and fitness is my life. If anyone understands the
importance of eating a healthy diet, it should be me. And what I know
for sure is that healthy eating and exercise go hand in hand. You can't
be successful with just one or the other. You need both. Exercise is fitness, and food is health. And we all want to be fit and healthy, right?
I'm going to say that again: *Exercise is fitness, and food is health.* I
want you to repeat that over and over until it sticks in your head like
a Maroon 5 song that won't go away. It sounds simple, but too many
people forget it.

I was always a skinny kid, and like the rest of the country, I lived
on the two staples of the American diet. Not meat and potatoes. I'm
talking about the 1960s and '70s (and beyond) staples of the American
diet: fast food and processed food. Nasty! But once I started to work out
and gain muscle, I began to realize the importance of healthy eating.
Unfortunately, I never liked—or learned how—to cook. Before I met

Melissa Costello, I was eating Amy's frozen dinners or takeout from the closest local "healthy" restaurant—certainly not my best option, but I did it out of convenience. What can I say? I was a bachelor (not "*The* Bachelor," *a* bachelor). I knew that I needed to change my diet and eat a wider variety of fresh food if I wanted to be the healthiest I could possibly be. I had tried other chefs here and there, but their "healthy" food lacked texture and taste. I was determined to find someone who could make me delicious, scrumptious, healthy food.

I met Melissa, owner of Karma Chow, about four years ago through a mutual friend. This friend kept insisting that I hire Melissa to cook for me. I hemmed and hawed because at the time, I thought hiring a full-time chef was a bit . . . well . . . *decadent.*

One day I was planning a small, intimate dinner party and needed a chef, so I called Melissa and she agreed to cook. Once I tasted her food, I was hooked. The flavors were so rich, yet it was all healthy—nothing processed, no sugar, no gluten, and no tofu. I was immediately blown away and had to hire her on the spot to cook for me every week. I couldn't believe that food could taste so good and actually be good for me, too.

You may know this already, but it turns out that food tastes so much better when it doesn't come from a box, a bag, or the freezer section. Who knew? Melissa's food is so satisfying that I never feel as if I am missing anything from my diet. I exercise hard and I need all that nutrition to recover and to build and restore my (rippling) muscles. Yes, I take supplements to help with that, but I know that eating healthy, whole foods is the foundation that provides me with the nutrients and strength I need to stay fit.

Eating a vegetarian/vegan diet for seventeen years provided me with strength and energy, and the clear, focused mind that I needed for a six-day-a-week workout plan. I later chose to shift my diet to a mostly plant-based diet, adding in some wild fish, free-range chicken, and eggs every once in a while due to my wacky travel schedule and not always being able to find high-quality vegan food on the road. I spend hours in the gym every week, and I know that without all the fresh, nutritious food that Melissa makes, I would not be able to exercise as hard as I do and build the muscle I need.

Her recipes are simple, yet *delicioso*! She has so many classic dishes that resemble the "real" (i.e., fattier and higher-calorie) versions that I don't even miss my grandmother's meatballs. (Noni, if you're reading this from heaven, I didn't mean it. I love your meatballs. Please go back to playing bingo and we'll talk about it when I see you in fifty years.)

Melissa's food is clean and provides me with the fuel I need to sleep well, heal my body, and perform better every day. She has a true gift in the kitchen and can turn any dish into a delectable vegan creation. Every time she cooks for me, the smells that waft from my kitchen are out of this world. I know it's no coincidence that friends start popping by the house just as Melissa's food is ready. And, amazingly, they never seem to have dinner plans. Problem is, I have a hard time sharing my food, as I want it all to myself. Is that selfish? Turns out that saying, "Go home and eat your own food" tends to drive friends away. So now I have to choose which is more important to me: Ed Nicoletti or Enchilada Casserole? Scott Fifer or Strawberry Crème Mousse? Pam the Blam or Pad Thai? It's a tough decision, I tell ya, but if you see Scott, Ed, or Pam, tell them I think of them fondly and to come find me at the bingo table with Noni in fifty years. Maybe sixty years if I keep eating Melissa's healthy food . . .

—**Tony Horton**
*Creator of P90X®, Power 90®, and Power Half Hour®*

# Introduction

## The Journey to Plant-Based Eating, Optimal Health, and Vivacious Vitality

*I am quite certain* that if you have picked up this book, you are definitely interested in learning more about eating healthy. If so, I want to congratulate and commend you for your commitment to yourself, your family, and anyone else in your life that will benefit from this positive choice.

As a nutritionist, I have been fortunate to work with hundreds of clients as they embrace a plant-based lifestyle, whether they are doing so to lose weight, boost their performance, gain more energy, or be kinder to the planet. In revamping the pantries of people from all walks of life—from semipro athletes and high-powered executives to budding entrepreneurs and busy moms—there is one commonality: for many of them, the idea of eating healthy can feel overwhelming without having the proper tools or education. Most of my clients have many distractions: extraneously long to-do lists, unanswered texts and e-mails, and many other things that make healthy food preparation a challenge. Many of them feel so inconvenienced by preparing meals that they hit the closest drive-through, or they subsist on the latest diet of packaged foods because they can add up points and it's "easy."

This is why I created the recipes in this book to be simple and delicious. I want to show you that eating healthy doesn't have to be daunting or time-consuming. Almost all of the ingredients can be found at well-stocked supermarkets, your local health food store, Trader Joe's or Whole Foods, farmers' markets, or even online (see the Resources section). There are ways to eat healthy no matter what your budget or time constraints—and I will show you how!

Although this cookbook does not contain any meat, cheese, dairy, or animal products, I did not create it to turn you into a vegan or vegetarian. I created it to teach you that eating a whole-food, plant-based diet can help you feel healthier, find your natural body weight (if you need to), sleep better, live longer, and give you more energy, just to name a few of the benefits. Most of the recipes in this book are gluten free, refined sugar free, and contain minimally processed foods. I created it this way so that you can see for yourself how easy it is to create delicious dishes without using preseasoned, packaged, and processed foods.

To me, this way of life is about keeping it simple. There are many cookbooks out there that are in line with my philosophy of eating and living, yet the recipes tend to be overly complicated. My intention when I wrote this book was to "keep it simple" and "make it tasty." Some of the recipes contained here will take more time than others, but I think you will find that most of them are fairly simple to make and very easy to integrate into your busy lifestyle.

You will learn about foods you've never heard of and foods that you may have seen in the grocery store but didn't have a clue how to use or how to make them taste good! (Can you say "kale"?) You will start to feel more alive, your vitality will increase, and your body will begin to balance itself out and function properly in the form of effortless digestion, clearer skin, and deeper sleep. It's like resetting your whole system. And if you have high cholesterol, inflammation, and aches and pains, you can say good-bye to those as well!

I also want to remind you that eating clean and living a life of optimal health is about taking the time to plan your food, whether you have a family or are single. Anytime we learn something new, there is always a learning curve, so remember that *planning* and *practice* are the two important keys here. This is not about eating perfectly; this is about taking small steps each and every day for positive, long-lasting change that will result in a life of health, energy, vitality, and wellness! I am excited to begin this journey with you, because I have been there firsthand and I know the difference it has made in my life!

## My Journey to Plant-Based Eating

As a kid growing up, I ate nothing but processed foods that were high in sugar, fat, and salt. The cabinets in my childhood home were stocked with the latest, most colorful, overly sweet, crunchy boxed concoction or salty, greasy, oily chip we could find. My dad worked for a vending machine company, so we had candy at our fingertips 24/7. Pop-Tarts for breakfast, chips and hot dogs for lunch, and dinner was usually cooked by Mom, Dad, or Grandmom, which was my only saving grace, really. In between meals, I ate sugar, sugar, sugar. I would eat it first thing in the morning, in between meals, and before bed. I was addicted to sugar (although I didn't know it at the time).

Eating processed food was all my family knew. With the best of intentions my mom packed my lunch—usually some processed lunch meat on a tasty, white Italian roll made fresh at the local bakery accompanied by some form of crunchy, greasy goodness in a bag.

This was how I was raised. It's interesting to note: I was always *sick*. You name it, I had it: strep throat, pink eye (multiple times per year), asthma, migraines, and digestive issues. I had the whole gamut. Thankfully, I was extremely active as a kid. I played every sport you can imagine, both recreationally and in school: soccer, softball, field hockey, baseball with the boys (yes, I know), and basketball.

As I moved into my late teens and early twenties, I was sick of feeling sick all the time, but no one could connect the dots to the cause of my ailments. Like many young women, I started to struggle with body-image issues as well. I knew I needed to get healthy, but I also had an ulterior motive: having the perfect body. I jumped on the "fat-free" bandwagon, thinking I was doing well for my body. If the box said "lite" or "fat-free" on it, I bought it. This meant that I was ingesting even more processed foods, and little did I know, they were loaded with sugar and chemicals. In the pursuit of being thin, I'd skip meals and eat fat-free foods only. I spent hours at the gym vying to whittle down and sculpt the perfect body that all the *Sports Illustrated* girls had!

This was my struggle for many years, and during this process I realized that I still didn't feel well or healthy, even though I thought I was eating better. I began to research food and its effects on the body. I learned about processed foods and how harmful they are to the system. So I began to cut back on them, but not in a healthy way: I became a food Nazi! Everything I put into my mouth was scrutinized by my skinny-girl voice inside. At this point, I had a full-blown eating disorder, and every second I was obsessed with what I put—or didn't put—into my mouth. I knew this way of living was not healthy for me, yet I didn't know how to stop it.

As I neared my thirties, I knew that I needed to make some big changes in my relationship to food. I knew that if I kept going the way I was, I would end up really sick and this would be a lifelong battle. I got tired of the voices in my head telling me I was fat and out of control. I wanted to relate to food differently and in a healthy way. I wanted to feel good from the inside out and praise my body for all that it provided for me. It wasn't just about looking good anymore, even though that was an added bonus that came from eating healthy; it was about feeling really well, being healthy, and living a long, vital, and energetic life.

I have to say that my knowledge about eating healthily did not always come easy, and yet it was a natural progression, because as I ate healthier foods, I started to feel better. I began studying nutrition, which led me to teaching myself healthier ways to cook everyday foods. I knew that putting fresh, whole foods into my body would help me with my eating disorder because I would find my natural body weight and stop obsessing over being stick thin. My goal would be to be fit and vibrant for a lifetime. I cut back on white sugar, gluten, and other processed foods. As I learned more and more and felt better and better, I gradually cut out other foods, including chicken and eggs, because I realized that they didn't feel good in my body anymore. It took a lot of experimenting to find what worked for me. I am not advocating that you cut out all the foods that I did; I am suggesting that you really think about what you put into your body and how it serves you.

Do you make healthy choices for yourself on a daily basis? Do you really know what your body wants and needs? Do you listen to your body and give it what it's asking for? Eating healthily and being healthy is a lifestyle. It is a *choice* and it takes commitment: a choice to take care of yourself and to feel good; a choice to eat whole, unprocessed, plant-based foods that give you fuel instead of sapping the life out of you; a choice to educate your kids and learn as much as you can so that your probability of living a long, vital, and energized life is higher.

The old adage is true: "You are what you eat." When we eat crappy food, we feel crappy. When we eat good, healthy food, we feel good. My client and P90X™ creator Tony Horton says that you can control two things in your life: what you put into your mouth and how you move your body. I agree! With this book, I am going to help you with the first one by introducing you to some amazingly delicious yet healthy recipes that will make your taste buds come alive and dispel any misbeliefs about vegan foods being bland or boring.

## My Food Philosophy

I'm sure that many of you can relate to the issues I have talked about regarding food and eating. That is why this book is so important in assisting you with making better choices and changing your relationship to food. It will help you transition into a healthier lifestyle that will provide vitality, energy, natural body weight, and so much more.

### Dieting . . . Does It Really Work?

How many of you have gone on a diet just to realize it doesn't work? You lose a bunch of weight for a short period of time, only to gain back twice as much within a year or two. There is a high probability that you don't feel well in the process, and usually after a short period, you revert to unhealthy habits that don't serve you. There are more diets out there than I care to name, yet *not one of them* educates us on *how* to eat healthily. That's why I strongly believe that *dieting does not work*. I have coached dozens of clients who have participated in almost every diet known to man at some point in their life, only to come to me defeated and hoping that I can help them change their lifestyle through teaching them how to eat clean and healthily. They are finally ready to *learn* and to *make long-term changes* for optimum vitality, energy, and health.

### *Stop Counting and Start Listening*

Counting calories is one way that people think they can get healthy, but in fact, the act of counting calories can result in deprivation, over-eating, and a misperception about how food metabolizes in our bodies. Yes, calorie counting can be good for people who need to lose a significant amount of weight. They need calorie deprivation *and* exercise to trick their body in the interim, but that effect doesn't last long. In my opinion, calorie counting turns our food into an object versus what it really is—nourishment, fuel, and life. It disconnects us from our food and the benefit that healthy, whole foods have in our lives. Calorie counting can cause the body to go into starvation mode, which results in a slower metabolism and weight holding. Your body will not release weight because it is holding on to every ounce it has as a survival tactic.

When I work with my cleanse clients, many of whom are fitness fanatics, I challenge them to stop counting calories for thirty days. This is very uncomfortable to some because they feel that the act of counting calories is what has kept them lean, healthy, and in control, and to some extent it probably has. Yet what they discover is that when they let go of counting every morsel they put into their mouth, there is a newfound freedom with food, and they actually find their own natural balance by listening to what their body wants instead of what they think it should have. They also find that eating whole foods fills them up for longer periods of time, and they feel more satisfied, have more energy, and don't need to eat as much because the food is so high in nutrients! WOW . . . all this from eating whole foods! So if you are an obsessive calorie counter, I challenge you to give it up and start listening to your body and what it really needs and wants!

## The Great Food Disconnect

In today's society, most of us get from day to day by rushing from place to place. We eat on the run, in our cars, and standing over the kitchen sink (guilty!). We've become disconnected from our food. Many of us don't sit down as families any longer, let alone cook our meals at home, and when we do sit down with our families, there is always a TV running or some other electronic device distracting quality time. I've seen so many beautifully crafted kitchens in Los Angeles that go unused day in and day out because people are just simply too busy to cook and sit down with their families for a nourishing meal. When did everything else in our lives become more important than sitting with our families and eating a home-cooked, delicious, whole-food meal? This is an important basis for our children and teaches them that eating nutritious food is the key to a long, happy, and healthy life. This disconnection from our food has led us to obesity, heart disease, diabetes, and many other illnesses that are so prevalent in society today.

If you want to be truly healthy and full of vitality and energy, you must go back to your roots and adopt the attitude of generations that have gone before us. Our grandparents and great-grandparents ate from the land. They grew their own food or got it from the local farm stand on the corner. They ate whole, unprocessed foods that were comprised of one ingredient. There were no boxes, bags, or artificial flavorings or colorings to give our food the look and smell of perfection so that we'd buy it. Did you know that there is a certain brand of popular corn chips out there that has *forty-two* ingredients in it? And

I can't even pronounce most of the ingredients. When did chemicals and artificial colorings become the norm? When did we let go of caring enough about our bodies and our health to really monitor what we put into them? When did we forget that food is our friend and that it keeps us alive?

Now is the time when we must make different choices regarding what we put into our bodies. We must reconnect to our food and honor it as the source that keeps us alive, along with water, air, and sleep. It's time to slow down, sit down, and take time out of our busy lives to nourish ourselves so that we can get through each day with energy, vigor, and vitality. It's time to make healthy eating a priority in our lives so that we can be of service to ourselves and others. So to that end, I invite you to really investigate your relationship to food, how you have been feeding yourself and your family, and how you feel when you don't put good stuff into your body. It's time to commit to *you* and to take positive steps to change your health and your life!

## Kitchen & Pantry Essentials

Having the basic essentials on hand in your kitchen is key to enjoying the process of cooking and eating. It is also helpful to purge your kitchen of any appliances that may be broken or that you do not use anymore. Below is a list of my favorite kitchen essentials/tools that will help. You don't need to purchase them all at once; you can buy them in stages. The list starts with the most important tools first.

### Basic Kitchen Tools

**Knives:** If you want your cooking experience to be pleasant and easy, it's important to invest in one or two really good knives. Not only does it make it more pleasurable to chop and dice, it's important for your safety as well. Dull knives cause slippage and dreaded finger cuts. I love to have an eight-inch chef's knife (also known as a French knife or cook's knife) or seven-inch Santoku knife on hand, as well as a really good paring knife for peeling fruits and veggies and cutting small items. A serrated knife is also great to have for cutting breads and softer foods like fruits, tomatoes, avocados, and so on. It's also smart to invest in a good knife sharpener as well. I like to use a whetstone for the best sharpening. The honer that comes in most cutlery sets is not really a sharpener, but is used to keep small nicks off your knife. You should hone your knives every time you use them to keep them in tip-top shape. If you invest in a high quality knife, be sure you take good care of it by cleaning it immediately and storing it properly with a knife cover or in a slotted kitchen drawer. I recommend buying knives separately versus in a set, as most of the knives in a set are not always utilized and could be a waste of money. My favorite brands of knives are Henckels, Wusthof, Miyabi (for Santoku knives), and Shun Ken as they are made from high-quality steel and come with a warranty (see Resources section on where to buy). I also love a good ceramic paring knife, which you can find easily at Sur La Table or online (Kyocera or Kuhn Rikon are both high-quality brands).

**Cutting Boards:** Cutting boards are another must-have for a pleasant cooking experience. Bamboo cutting boards are the best, as they do not absorb bacteria like plastic cutting boards do. It's good to have various sizes so you don't have to lug out a large cutting board if you only need to chop one sprig of cilantro.

**Cookware & Bakeware:** It's really important to invest in quality cookware when you can. You are on the road to healthy eating, and having proper cookware will support that. Nonstick and aluminum cookware can be toxic due to the release of harmful chemicals when heated, so it's best to get rid of these types of cookware if you have them. Stainless steel is the best, and although it's a bit expensive, it will literally last you a lifetime. All-Clad is my favorite brand, and they guarantee their products for life! Cast-iron pans are really good as well, and there are many brands available. Le Creuset makes great cast-iron pots and pans that are beautiful and will last a lifetime. Last, if you are really attached to your nonstick cookware, there are a few companies that make "green" nonstick cookware that I personally find very useful for browning or cooking certain foods, such as pancakes or veggie burgers, without the worry of them sticking.

Here are some basics to get you started: soup or stock pot, 3-quart saucepan with a lid, 12-inch skillet with a lid, 10-inch sauté pan, and a 10-inch nonstick "green" skillet. It's also good to have a variety of glass or ceramic casserole dishes, especially since there are a lot of casserole-type recipes in this book.

It's also nice to have various types of bakeware in your kitchen so that you can whip up healthy desserts. Here are a few ideal pieces: a loaf pan, a muffin pan, a mini muffin pan (for Banana Chocolate Chip Minis or Black Bean Brownie Bites; see recipes on pages 29 and 195), a springform pan (for Luscious Limey "Cheese"cake; see recipe on page 217), an 8 × 8-inch cake pan, and baking sheets for cookies.

**Peelers, Strainers & Graters:** All of these items are extremely helpful in a kitchen, and you might use them on a daily basis or every time you cook. Having a quality peeler is really important to efficiently peel fresh veggies. Fine-sieve strainers and colanders are lifesavers in my kitchen. It's good to have at least one large colander for draining pasta, potatoes, and larger items. Fine-sieve strainers are essential for rinsing grains and beans. I use a variety of sizes, even a tiny one for straining lemon seeds or tea leaves from my homemade chai (see recipe for Divine Coconutty Chai on page 51). Graters or zesters are also helpful tools in your plant-based kitchen. Microplanes are my favorite as they are simple to use and will zest or grate anything from garlic to nutmeg! A citrus reamer is also great to have for "squeezing" citrus fruits.

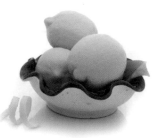

**Spatulas, Wooden Spoons & Other Helpful Utensils:** It's wise to have a variety of wooden spoons for mixing and stirring, silicone spatulas that will withstand high heat, tongs for easy grasping, and a flat spatula for turning meatless patties and pancakes.

**Mixing Bowls & Prep Bowls:** There is nothing more satisfying to me than cutting up a bunch of colorful, fresh veggies for a soup, stir-fry, or stew and putting them in glass prep bowls. I then line them up as I'm ready to start cooking, and it's so easy to grab each ingredient as I need it, and it's colorful, too! Buying a variety of prep bowls will be really helpful to you, especially if you are new to the kitchen. I also make sure I have a variety of glass or stainless mixing bowls for baking, tossing salads, or soaking grains and beans.

**Salad Spinner:** This is a must-have in my kitchen since I eat so many greens. I highly recommend that you buy one, too. They are not expensive, and they are so great for soaking and cleaning your greens before storing them.

**Coffee Grinder:** Not just for coffee anymore, this can grind spices, nuts, and seeds in a snap. You can find one for about $10 at a drugstore.

**Mortar & Pestle:** These are helpful for hand-grinding seeds, herbs, and spices, not to mention how cute they look on the kitchen counter. You can find them cheap at any department store or TJ Maxx–type discount store.

## Other Helpful Items

**Food Processor:** This is a really smart investment for a plant-based kitchen, but if you are not ready to purchase a large food processor, go with a mini version or a combination processor/blender. A food processor is great for making dips, spreads, and sauces, so it really is a key kitchen tool. Cuisinart is my favorite brand; it comes with a good warranty and a variety of cup sizes.

**Blender or Vitamix:** Having a good blender in your kitchen is essential. In my opinion, Vitamix is the best and a great investment. You can make soups, nut butters, smoothies, and so much more in a Vitamix. Yes, they are expensive, but they are worth the price when you are ready, and they will last for many years to come!

**Magic Bullet:** This little appliance chops, blends, and mixes. It also comes with a blender attachment, so is very convenient for making smoothies.

**Rice Cooker:** This will definitely simplify the process of cooking your grains. Just measure out the grains and water, pour in the cooker, cover with a lid, turn it on, and walk away. You will have delicious cooked grains in about twenty minutes.

**Pressure Cooker:** This is useful for cooking soups and beans in a flash. I must confess: I've lived without one of these most of my cooking life, but some chefs swear by them. They will cut your bean cooking time in half and help your grains stay moist.

**Glass Jars:** These are handy to use to store grains, nuts, seeds, and legumes, and to keep your kitchen organized. I love seeing lines of jars in my kitchen full of colorful beans, grains, and nuts.

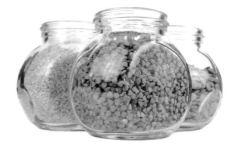

# Healthy Pantry Must-Haves

I've included a basic "shopping list" of my favorite grains, legumes, nuts, spices, herbs, condiments, and oils to have on hand. You can always add to this list, but these are the basic staples. I know you may not be familiar with some of the foods listed below, but it's good to step outside of what you know and try new things. I have never had a client of mine dislike any of my suggestions (okay, maybe once or twice). Most of these items can be found at any natural food store. You can also order things like oils, spices, dried beans, and other items online (see the Resources section). I will also talk more about some of these foods as they are listed in certain recipes.

| Grains | Legumes | Nuts/Seeds | Vinegars | Oils |
|---|---|---|---|---|
| Barley | Adzuki beans | Raw almonds | Apple cider | Almond oil |
| Brown basmati and jasmine rice | Black beans | Cashews | Balsamic | Avocado oil |
| Buckwheat | Cannellini beans | Flax, chia, and hemp seeds | Brown rice | Coconut oil |
| Millet | Great Northern White Beans | Pecans | Champagne | Flaxseed oil |
| Quinoa | Chickpeas | Pine nuts | Mirin | Grapeseed oil |
| Short-grain brown rice | Kidney beans | Pumpkin seeds | Raspberry | Extra virgin olive oil |
| Steel-cut or rolled oats | Lentils: green and red | Sesame seeds | Red wine | Sesame oil |
| Wheat berries | Split peas | Sunflower seeds | Sherry | Walnut oil |
| Wild rice | | Walnuts | Umeboshi | |

## Beans: Buying in Bulk or in a Can?

Buying beans in bulk and cooking them at home will provide these positive results versus buying canned beans:

1. Saves money
2. Less gas and bloating
3. More nutritional value
4. Saves time by bulk cooking and freezing
5. Less sodium

### How Do I Cook My Beans?

Using a pressure cooker is best, but a regular old pot will do, too. Soak the beans overnight in a pot of cold water with a 1-inch piece of kombu. Kombu is a sea vegetable, also known as kelp, and is found in the international aisle of most markets (see Resources section). Soaking the beans with kombu helps them to become more easily digestible and cuts back on the gas-inducing properties. If you cannot find kombu, just go without; you will still get nearly the same benefit from soaking. In the morning, drain the water and rinse the beans really well. Put back into the pot with the kombu and fill with cold water about 2 inches above the beans. Turn heat to high and bring to a boil. Scrape the foam off the top, and then lower the heat to simmer. Cook for 1 to 3 hours depending on the type of bean. The bigger the bean, the longer it takes to cook. (Also, the bigger the bean, the more gas they provide.) Once tender, drain and store in the refrigerator or freeze for later use; you can keep them frozen for one month in a tightly sealed container or freezer bag.

# Spices & Herbs

These are some of my favorite spices and herbs:

## Spices

| | | | |
|---|---|---|---|
| Black peppercorns | Cinnamon | Fennel seeds | Paprika |
| Cardamom | Cloves | Garam masala | Sea salt |
| Chili powder | Coriander | Ginger | Tarragon |
| Chipotle chili powder | Cumin | Mustard seeds | |
| | Curry powder | Nutmeg | |

## Herbs *(You can purchase any of these either dried or fresh.)*

| | | |
|---|---|---|
| Basil | Marjoram | Parsley |
| Bay leaves | Mint | Rosemary |
| Dill | Oregano | Thyme |

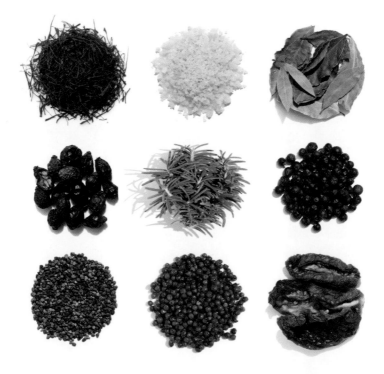

**Agave or fruit-juice sweetened ketchup:** Most brands of ketchup are loaded with sugar, but agave or fruit-juice sweetened ketchup is a really tasty alternative that won't give you the blood sugar spike.

**Bragg's Aminos:** This soy sauce alternative is good to use in place of the high-sodium condiment. It's loaded with amino acids and protein.

**Dairy-free milks:** almond, cashew, coconut, hemp, multigrain, oat, and rice. Nut milks are easy to make on your own, but if you don't have the time, you can easily find them in your grocery store. These are all great alternatives to dairy, but be sure to buy unsweetened, as they can contain a lot of unnecessary sugar.

## CHEF'S TIP: A WORD ABOUT SOY

Soy comes in many forms. You will not find any tofu or soy milk in my cookbook, as I find it to be overly processed and disruptive to the digestive and hormonal system. The only types of soy products I use are the actual soybean itself (also known as edamame) and miso, tamari, and tempeh, which are all fermented and therefore gentler and healthier for the system. Make sure to always buy organic soy, as it tends to be one of the most genetically modified crops in the United States. Tempeh is a high-protein meat substitute that contains soybeans fermented with grain. It tends to be easier to digest than tofu for most people, and I like its meaty texture. It also takes on the flavor of whatever it's cooked with, so it's very versatile. Miso is fermented soybean paste, which is used in dressing, soups, and sauces, and is very alkalizing for the body. The Japanese typically eat miso soup every day for breakfast to alkalize their systems as they "break their fast." Tamari is a type of soy sauce that is usually wheat free and fermented and can be used in any dish that calls for soy sauce.

**Dijon mustard and stone-ground mustard:** I love to have both of these in my fridge for adding zip and thickness to dressings.

**Earth Balance Natural Buttery Spread (soy free):** A healthier alternative to trans-fatty margarines and butter (also gluten and dairy free).

**Ener-G Egg Replacer:** This is a product made from potato starch, tapioca starch flour, and nondairy leavening (it is also low/no sodium, low protein, and contains no nuts, wheat, gluten, casein, yeast, egg, soy, or dairy). It comes in powder form and is whisked with water to replace eggs in recipes.

**Gluten-free pastas or sprouted grain pastas:** These are still considered processed, so eat them only a couple of times a week. There are so many delicious alternatives out there now to high-glycemic white flour and processed pasta, so be creative and try out a few different brands to see what you like best.

**Gluten-free & sprouted grain breads/tortillas/bread crumbs:** My favorites include Food for Life Brown Rice Tortillas and breads, Ezekiel Sprouted-Grain Tortillas and breads, and Glutino breads, which are great for vegetarians (most are not vegan). Some of my favorite gluten-free bread mixes are Bob's Red Mill, Namaste Foods, and Gluten Free Pantry.

**Mellow white miso or any miso:** Miso is great for dressings, sauces, and stir-fry. I especially like the mellow white as it's a bit on the sweet side and not as strong as a barley or brown rice miso.

**Nut & seed butters:** These include almond, cashew, peanut, pumpkin seed, and sunflower. These are staples in my pantry for extra protein and healthy fats. Be sure to buy unsweetened or read the label for added sugar.

**Nutritional yeast flakes:** You can find these in the supplement section of your health food market. Many vegans rely on nutritional yeast for their B vitamins. I love it for its cheesy flavor (you'll probably notice

I use it a lot in recipes as an alternative to cheese).

**Sea Salt:** It's best to use sea salt instead of table salt as it's higher in minerals and less processed. It will help to restore a healthy balance in your body versus depleting it like regular table salt can do. Himalayan pink salt is the best, but if you can't find that, my next favorite is Real Salt straight from Utah.

**So Delicious Coconut Creamer (Unsweetened):** This is my latest obsession. I love it in my morning green tea.

**Tamari (low sodium):** Tamari is usually a wheat-free version of soy sauce. Make sure to buy low sodium.

**Tempeh:** Nutty with a meaty texture, tempeh is fermented with grains and is a wonderful addition to chili or to any recipe where you would normally use meat. It's loaded with protein and is much easier to digest than its jiggly counterpart, tofu.

**Vegan Worcestershire sauce:** Made without anchovies, it is easily found in any health food store.

**Vegenaise (Grapeseed Oil or Soy Free):** Vegenaise is a healthy, vegan alternative to mayo with lots of flavor. You can find it in the refrigerator section in any health food market.

**Xanthan gum:** This is added to most gluten-free flours to add elasticity to baked goods in vegan cooking, and it is also used in some sauces and dressings. Most vegan chefs like it because it is tasteless and odorless. It is pricey ($10 to $12 for 8 ounces), but since recipes call for such a small amount, it's worth it. You can store it in the fridge to preserve it.

## What About Baking?

Gone are the days of vegan baked goods that have the consistency of a brick. There are so many gluten-free, healthy whole grain flours available, as well as alternative sweeteners, that it is truly simple and fun to whip up delicious baked goods without the guilt. Below is a list of some of my favorites that I use in my baking and everyday cooking.

**Flours:** You can use the flours listed for a variety of different foods. I like to use a combination of flours when baking cookies, cakes, and other baked goods because it adds different textures and flavors. It's fun to experiment, but keep in mind that gluten-free flours don't bake the same way white flour does. You will need to add xanthan gum to most gluten-free flours to provide the "glue" that gluten usually provides. (See "Baking Substitutions 101" at the back of the book for exact amounts of alternative flours to substitute for white flour.)

| | | |
|---|---|---|
| Almond flour/meal | Brown rice flour | Millet flour |
| Bob's Red Mill Gluten Free All Purpose Baking Flour | Buckwheat flour | Oat flour |
| | Chickpea flour | Spelt flour |
| | Coconut flour | |

### The Glycemic Index

The glycemic index (GI) is a numerical scale used to indicate how quickly and how high a particular food can raise our blood glucose levels. Foods that are lower on the glycemic index are better for our blood sugar levels and do not give us the highs and lows that high-glycemic foods can. For a complete list of foods and their GI count, check out http://www.glycemicindex.com/.

### Alternative Sweet Stuff

**Blackstrap Molasses:** Blackstrap molasses has a deep, rich flavor and it's loaded with minerals, including potassium, magnesium, calcium, and iron.

**Brown rice syrup:** This has a malty, mellow flavor and is the least sweet of all the alternative sweeteners. Be sure to buy an organic brown rice syrup.

**Coconut palm sugar (organic):** A granular brown sugar that is made from the sap and nectar of coconut palm trees, this sweetener contains B and C vitamins and is high in potassium, magnesium, zinc, and iron. It is great for baking.

**Dark Raw Blue Agave Nectar:** Extracted from the agave plant, agave nectar is 1.3 times sweeter than sugar, so you don't need to use as much in your recipes.

**Grade B maple syrup:** This is a lower glycemic sweetener that is derived from the sap of the maple tree.

**Lakanto:** A crystallized sugar made from erythritol, which is a fermented sugar alcohol from the lo han guo fruit, this sweetener has zero effect on your blood sugar levels and is good for preventing tooth decay.

**Stevia:** This is a sweetener that is 300 times sweeter than sugar and is made from the stevia plant. It's good to use for sweetening dressings and drinks. You can also use it for baking, but it doesn't provide the best consistency or flavor for baked goods. It comes in powdered or liquid form, but it's better to use in its most natural form. Be wary of powdered stevia with additives. As an alternative to packaged stevia, you can buy a stevia plant, grind up the leaves, and add it to your tea.

## Find Your Fun in the Kitchen

Now that you have your pantry stocked and your kitchen ready to go, it's time to cook. Cooking should not feel like a chore you have to do. If you picked up this book, you're probably interested in eating healthy for the long-term, so my suggestion is that you gradually integrate healthy cooking into part of your lifestyle toward optimal health and wellness. When you eat out, you cannot control what goes into your food, even if you think it's healthy.

Planning is going to be the number one key to your healthy life. And when I say planning, I mean sitting down and writing down the foods you want to eat for the week and then making a plan to buy and cook them. You don't have to go crazy, but make three or four simple dishes and keep them stored in the fridge for ease, especially after a long day at work.

One thing I really enjoy doing when I cook is to turn my vegetable chopping into a meditation of sorts. I turn on some good music, sharpen my knife, get out my large cutting board and glass bowls, and go to town. I love to smell all the fresh veggies, feel their textures in my hands, and revel at all the amazing colors that the earth can provide for our bodies. I chop away and put all my cut-up veggies in different bowls and then get to see all the beautiful colors together! When I'm done with all that chopping, I'm ready to assemble all the ingredients to create a satisfying and delicious dish.

Working with fresh whole foods inspires me, whereas eating foods that come from a box or a bag and are produced in a factory just doesn't feel as good. Yes, it may be quicker, but is it really as nourishing and healthy for me as all the fresh, beautiful foods I can get at the local farmer's market or grocery store? No way!

So as you go into your kitchen, I want you to keep all this in mind. Most of us love food that tastes good, and when we cook it ourselves we get to put so much love and positive energy into it, as well as be grateful for all the nutrition and fuel it provides for our bodies. So have some fun, sharpen your knives, turn on the music, and let's get cooking!

# Chapter 1

# *Plant-Based Breakfasts and Beverages*

*B*reakfast is the most important meal of the day, yet many of us skip it or opt for coffee and a banana. Eating a nutritious breakfast that's high in fiber, complex carbs, and protein will rev up your metabolism and give you the fuel you need to get through your day. The recipes here are delicious, simple to make, and animal free, so you won't feel bogged down with heavy food first thing in the morning. While I included the smoothies in the breakfast section, you can enjoy them as great pick-me-up any time of the day.

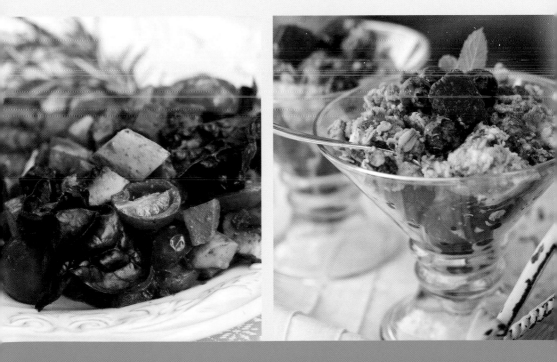

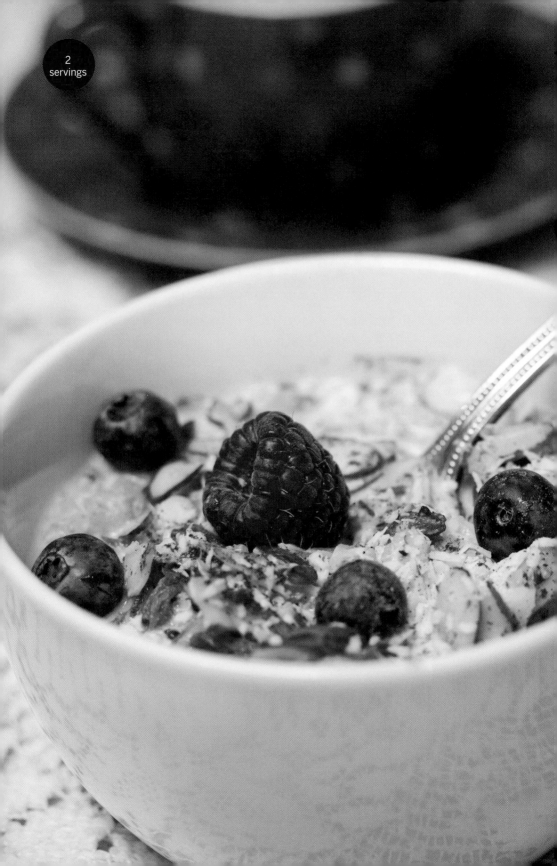

# Quinoa Protein Brekkie Bowl

*This breakfast bowl is loaded with protein and is an
awesome way to start your day. Kids love this, too, and it will keep
them going through a school day without that midmorning slump.
You can eat this warm or cold; either way, it's super delish!*

Cook the quinoa on a stovetop per package directions (or cook 1 cup quinoa in a rice cooker with 2 cups water).

While the quinoa is cooking, heat the oven to 350 degrees F. Spread the coconut and almonds on an ungreased, rimmed baking sheet and bake for 5 to 10 minutes, stirring once or twice, until golden brown. Remove from the oven.

When the quinoa is done cooking, add the coconut, almonds, raisins, hemp seeds, cardamom, cinnamon, agave nectar, and salt, and mix together. Top with almond or coconut milk to your liking and add fresh berries.

1 cup rinsed quinoa

¼ cup toasted, unsweetened coconut flakes

¼ cup toasted slivered almonds

¼ cup golden raisins

2 tablespoons hemp seeds

Pinch cardamom

1 teaspoon cinnamon

1 tablespoon agave nectar or maple syrup

Dash sea salt

Unsweetened almond milk or coconut milk, to taste

Optional: fresh berries

**Karmic Health Tip:** *This breakfast bowl is great made with millet, which is also high in protein and tonifying for your kidneys.*

Per Serving: Calories 520, Total Fat 22g, Sat. Fat 7g, Cholesterol 0mg, Sodium 20mg, Carbohydrate 70g, Fiber 10g, Protein 16g

**CHEF'S TIP: HOW TO MAKE FLAXSEED EGGS**

Several of the breakfast recipes call for flaxseed eggs. These are easy to make and a really good substitution for real eggs. To make two flaxseed eggs, combine 2 tablespoons of ground flaxseed with 6 tablespoons of water in a blender and blend until gelatinous. Let it sit in the fridge for 5 minutes to gel even more. (Use half of the ingredients to make one flaxseed egg.)

# Apricot Tea Muffins

Makes
16–18
muffins

*I love muffins in the morning. These muffins are gluten free and light, and delicious to have with a cup of tea. Try them with my homemade Divine Coconutty Chai (page 51) and you will be in breakfast heaven!*

Preheat the oven to 350 degrees F. Line a 12-muffin tin with paper liners or grease with coconut oil. In a medium-size bowl, whisk together the flour, baking powder, baking soda, xanthan gum, salt, cinnamon, and nutmeg.

In another bowl whisk together the coconut oil, apricot spread, agave nectar, almond milk, vanilla, and egg replacer. Add the wet ingredients to the dry and beat with a wooden spoon or use a hand mixer. When the batter is smooth and slightly sticky, add in the chopped apricots and stir to combine. Place the batter into the muffin cups about two-thirds full. Bake in the center of the oven for 18 to 20 minutes or until firm (test with a wooden toothpick). Place the muffin pan on a rack to cool slightly. Remove the muffins when slightly cooled and continue cooling on a wire rack to avoid sogginess. Store in an airtight container for up to three days.

1½ cups Bob's Red Mill Gluten-Free Flour

1½ teaspoons baking powder

1 teaspoon baking soda

1 teaspoon xanthan gum

½ teaspoon sea salt

1 teaspoon cinnamon

½ teaspoon nutmeg

⅓ cup coconut oil, melted (run the jar under hot water to melt the oil)

½ cup apricot spread, fruit only (no sugar added)

⅓ cup agave nectar

½ cup almond milk

2 teaspoons vanilla extract

Ener-G Egg Replacer for 2 eggs (whisked with warm water) or 2 flaxseed eggs

½ cup chopped, dried apricots

**Karmic Health Tip:** *Did you know that white sugar is not really vegan? It is processed with ash made from animal bone, so make sure if you are going to use sugar that you buy vegan sugar or some other less-processed version (see "Alternative Sweet Stuff" on page 20).*

Per Serving: Calories 140, Total Fat 4.5g, Saturated Fat 3.5g, Cholesterol 0mg, Sodium 430mg, Carbohydrate 24g, Fiber 1g, Protein 2g

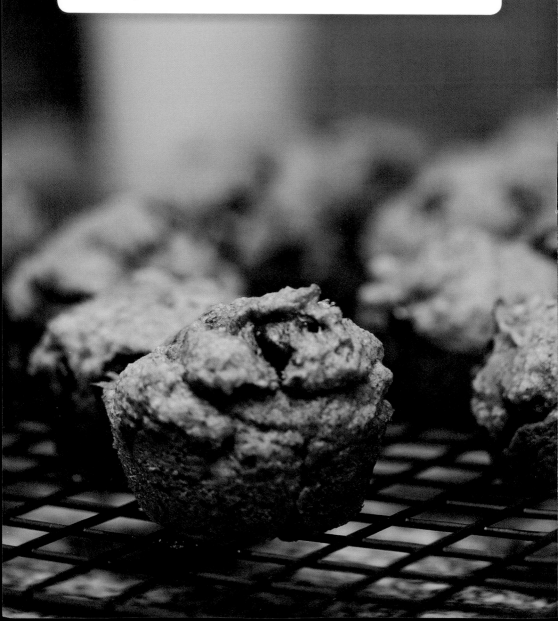

# Banana Chocolate Chip Minis

30–32
mini
muffins

*My sister-in-law loves to cook healthy food for her two-year-old, so she challenged me to make a more nutritious version of her banana chocolate chip muffin recipe, and these are the result. Even though they have chocolate in them, they are still nutritious enough to eat for breakfast.*

Preheat the oven to 350 degrees F. Line mini muffin tins with papers or grease with coconut oil.

In a large bowl, stir together the flour, baking soda, salt, cinnamon, and cardamom (if using). In a smaller bowl, whisk together the coconut oil and agave nectar until well combined. Add the flaxseed eggs, banana, and vanilla, and stir together until well incorporated.

Pour the banana mixture over the dry mix and stir with a wooden spoon to combine well. Stir in the chocolate chips. Fill mini muffin tins about two-thirds full. Bake for 7 to 10 minutes. Remove from the oven and place on a wire rack to cool. These can keep up to five days in an airtight container.

2 cups oat flour or spelt flour

1½ teaspoons baking soda

½ teaspoon salt

¼ teaspoon cinnamon

¼ teaspoon cardamom (optional)

½ cup coconut oil, melted, or grapeseed oil

½ cup agave nectar or maple syrup or 1 cup date puree

2 flaxseed eggs

3 ripe bananas, mashed

2 teaspoons vanilla

½ cup vegan or grain-sweetened chocolate chips

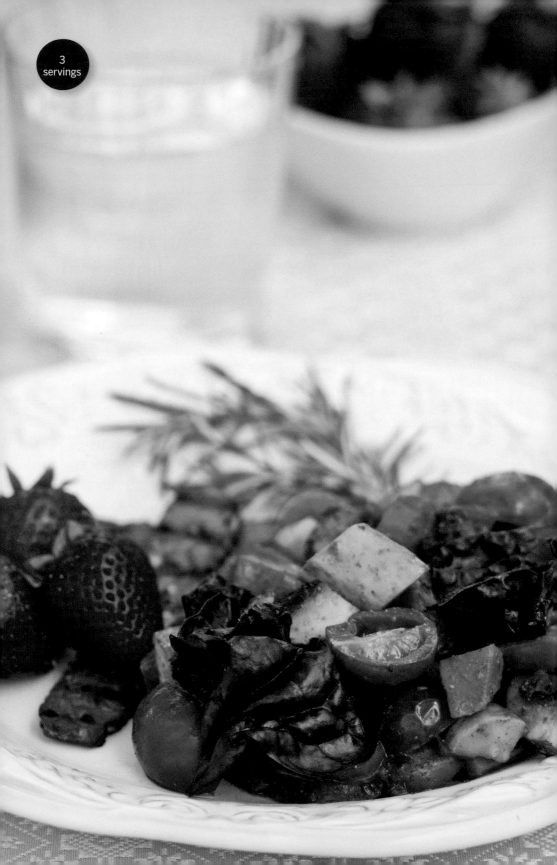

# Veggie Breakfast Scramble

*Most plant-based breakfast scrambles are made with overly processed tofu. I decided to give you a healthier version that is just as satisfying. Wrap it up in a sprouted grain or gluten-free tortilla for an "eggless" breakfast burrito or eat it alongside the delicious Tempeh Sausage Patties (page 35).*

Heat the olive oil in a large skillet over medium heat and sauté the peppers, mushrooms, onion, and garlic until soft and caramelized. Add the yams, cumin, paprika, tamari, and water. Cover the skillet and let the yams steam until soft, about 7 minutes. Add the tomatoes, zucchini, squash, and nutritional yeast and stir well to combine. Cook for another 7 minutes or until the veggies are soft, but not mushy. Add the chard and cover to wilt down, about 3 minutes. Serve immediately.

2 tablespoons olive oil

1 green bell pepper, diced

½ red bell pepper, diced

10 mushrooms, thinly sliced

½ medium red onion, diced

1 teaspoon minced garlic

1 garnet yam, peeled and cut into ¼-inch cubes

1 teaspoon cumin

½ teaspoon paprika

1 tablespoon tamari

1 tablespoon water

½ cup halved cherry tomatoes

1 cup diced zucchini

½ cup diced yellow squash

3 tablespoons nutritional yeast

1 cup Swiss chard, torn into pieces

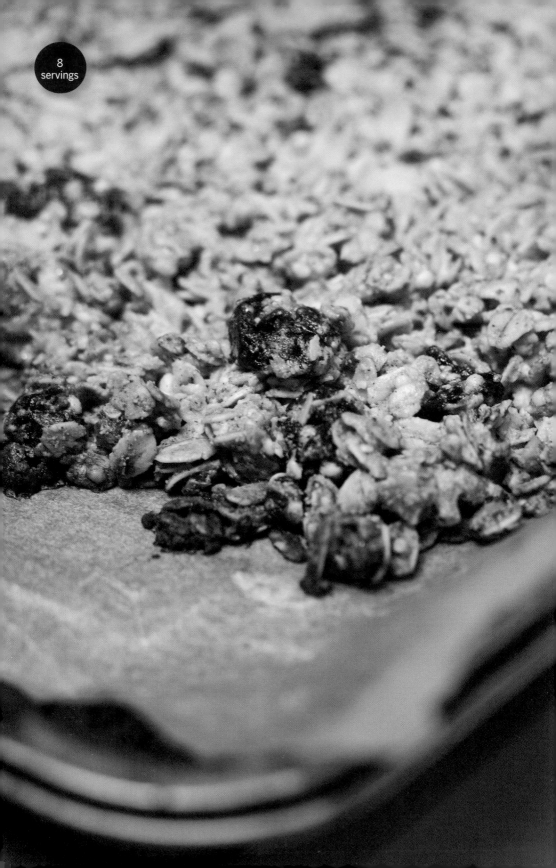

8
servings

# Karmic Cherry Almond Granola

*Granola is an awesome staple for breakfast. It's great to
make a couple of batches of this on a weekend and store it in an
airtight container to eat anytime you feel like you want a healthy,
nutritious snack or breakfast. It's also a key ingredient
in my Rise and Shine Granola Parfaits (page 39).*

Preheat the oven to 350 degrees
F. Combine the oats, flour, almonds,
cherries, hemp seeds, salt, cinnamon,
and cardamom in a large mixing bowl
and mix well. In a separate small bowl,
whisk the coconut oil, maple syrup,
and vanilla until well combined. Pour
the wet ingredients over the dry and
stir well to combine. Place on a baking sheet lined with parchment paper
and spread it out evenly. Bake until it's
golden brown, approximately 30 min
utes. Remove the pan from the oven
and let the granola sit for 5 minutes
until it's crispy, then break into small
chunks. Once cooled, place in an airtight container.

3 cups rolled oats, not instant

1 cup oat flour or spelt flour

1 cup chopped almonds or any
other nut

½ cup chopped dried cherries

½ cup hemp seeds

½ teaspoon sea salt

½ teaspoon cinnamon

½ teaspoon cardamom

¾ cup coconut oil, melted

¾ cup maple syrup or agave
nectar

1 teaspoon vanilla or almond
extract, alcohol free if
available

**Did You Know?** Tempeh is a high-protein meat substitute consisting of soybeans that have been fermented with grains, such as rice or millet. Fermenting makes tempeh easier to digest than tofu, it's higher in nutrients, and it's less processed as well. Tempeh can be crumbled, cubed, marinated, baked, or steamed; it's as versatile a protein as they come and takes on the flavor of whatever it's cooked with.

## CHEF'S TIP

Steaming tempeh for about 7 minutes before cooking it can release the bitter flavor it may sometimes have. I like to use Lightlife brand, which tends to be the least bitter of all the brands, and it offers a wide variety of flavors, too, such as veggie, flax, and wild rice.

# Tempeh Sausage Patties

*Who needs real artery-clogging sausage when you can have flavorful Tempeh Sausage Patties without all the fat and calories of processed patties? Serve them alongside my Buckwheat Corn Cakes with Blueberry Drizzle (page 37).*

Combine the tempeh cubes with the vegetable broth and salt in a medium-size saucepan over medium heat. Bring the mixture to a boil, lower the heat, and simmer for 20 minutes or until the tempeh is moist. Remove the tempeh from the heat and drain into a colander. Pour it into a large bowl.

Meanwhile, warm 1 tablespoon of the olive oil in a medium-size skillet over medium heat. Add the onion, garlic, and red pepper flakes. Cook for approximately 7 minutes, until the onions are softened, stirring occasionally. Add the sage, thyme, and fennel seeds, and cook for 2 more minutes to release the flavor of the herbs. Remove the mixture from the heat and add it to the tempeh. Add the chickpea flour and, using your hands, combine the mixture together. Form the mixture into sixteen equal-sized balls, then press firmly into patties that are approximately 2 inches in diameter. In a heavy medium-size skillet, preferably nonstick, heat the remaining tablespoon of olive oil. Add the patties and cook until browned, approximately 3 minutes per side; remove the patties to a plate. Repeat with the remaining patties, adding a touch more oil to the pan if needed. Serve immediately.

2 8-ounce packages tempeh, cut into ¼-inch cubes

2 cups vegetable broth

1 teaspoon sea salt

2 tablespoons extra virgin olive oil

1 small yellow onion, finely chopped

2 cloves garlic, minced

½ teaspoon red pepper flakes

2 teaspoons dried sage

2 teaspoons dried thyme

1 teaspoon fennel seeds

¼ to ½ cup chickpea or garbanzo bean flour

Per Serving: Calories 80, Total Fat 5g, Saturated Fat 1g, Cholesterol 0mg, Sodium 200mg, Carbohydrate 5g, Fiber 1g, Protein 6g

# Buckwheat Corn Cakes with Blueberry Drizzle

*I love pancakes, but I didn't always like how heavy they felt in my belly. This lighter, gluten-free version is great with Blueberry Drizzle!*

| | |
|---|---|
| ½ cup buckwheat flour | 1½ cups almond or rice milk |
| ¾ cup fine cornmeal | ¼ cup water |
| ¼ cup ground chia seeds | 1 teaspoon cinnamon |
| 2 teaspoons baking powder | ½ ripe banana, mashed |
| ¼ teaspoon sea salt | 1 tablespoon melted coconut oil |

In a large bowl mix together all of the ingredients through the banana. Heat the coconut oil on a nonstick griddle over medium heat. Once the griddle is hot, pour the batter onto the griddle using a ¼ cup of the corn cake mixture. Cook over medium heat until bubbly and brown. Flip over and cook on the other side for a few minutes until brown. Serve with the Blueberry Drizzle (recipe follows) or your choice of topping.

Per Serving: Calories 130, Total Fat 4g, Saturated Fat 1.5g, Cholesterol 0mg, Sodium 180mg, Carbohydrate 22g, Fiber 4g, Protein 3g

## Blueberry Drizzle

| | |
|---|---|
| 1½ tablespoons arrowroot or kuzu root starch | 3 tablespoons maple syrup |
| ½ cup water or apple juice | 1 teaspoon vanilla |
| 2 cups frozen wild blueberries | Juice and zest of 1 lemon (the zest is the secret ingredient) |

Dissolve the arrowroot in the water and set aside. In a small saucepan over medium heat, add the blueberries, arrowroot mixture, maple syrup, vanilla, lemon juice, and lemon zest. Cook until thickened, while stirring continuously. Serve warm over pancakes.

Per Serving: Calories 50, Total Fat 0g, Saturated Fat 0g, Cholesterol 0mg, Sodium 0mg, Carbohydrate 13g, Fiber 1g, Protein 0g

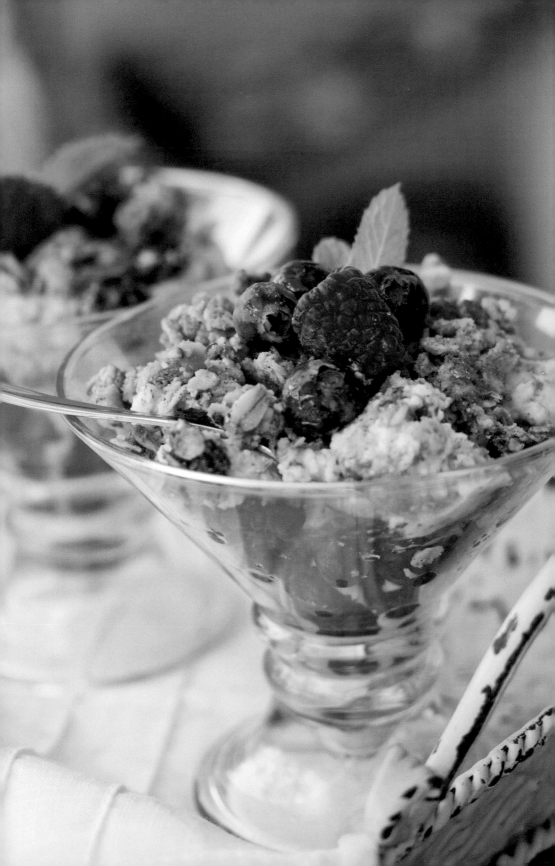

# Rise and Shine
# Granola Parfaits

*Parfaits are colorful, fun, and loaded with nutrients.
Use any kind of berries you want, and if berries aren't in season,
use apples, kiwi, banana, or whatever fruit you can find. No matter
what your fruit combo, these are simply divine in the morning.*

Divide the fruit among six wine or parfait glasses, layering each on top of the other, alternating red with blue. Spoon the Frangipane Crème over the berries and then add a thin layer of granola. Add another layer of berries. Add a dollop of Frangipane Crème, top with granola, and a drizzle of agave nectar (if you like) and a dash of cinnamon on each. Serve immediately.

2 pints fresh strawberries, hulled and quartered

1 pint fresh blueberries

1 pint fresh raspberries

1 cup Raw Almond Frangipane Crème (page 203)

1 cup Karmic Cherry Almond Granola (page 33)

Drizzle of agave nectar (optional)

Dash of cinnamon

# Cold Cinnamon Oaty Cereal

*So many of us eat hot cereal for breakfast, but I have clients
who love cold cereal in the morning, so I created this special dish for them.
Soaking the oats overnight gives them a pleasingly chewy texture.
Just add any kind of fruit you like and you have a really delightful
cold cereal that is nutritious and not processed.*

½ cup steel-cut oats

1 cup almond or coconut milk

1 teaspoon cinnamon

¼ teaspoon nutmeg

1 tablespoon chopped walnuts

2 teaspoons agave nectar or
maple syrup

¼ cup fresh blueberries or
strawberries

Soak the oats in the refrigerator overnight for at least ten hours in the almond or coconut milk. Add the remaining ingredients and serve cold.

# Cashew Milk

*I love to make my own raw milk. It's so easy, as you can see here.
Double the batch and keep it in your fridge to eat with
cereal or granola, to use in smoothies, or
wherever you would use milk.*

Drain the water from the cashews.
Place all of the ingredients in a
blender cup and blend until smooth.
If you want a creamier consistency,
you can strain the milk with a fine
sieve strainer or through cheesecloth.

1 cup raw cashews, soaked for 2 hours

1 tablespoon raw agave nectar

1 teaspoon vanilla extract

Dash sea salt

4 cups filtered water or coconut water
 (for a sweeter milk)

Dash cinnamon

Dash nutmeg

## CHEF'S TIP

Use this recipe for any type of nut milk. Just swap out the cashews for your
nut of choice.

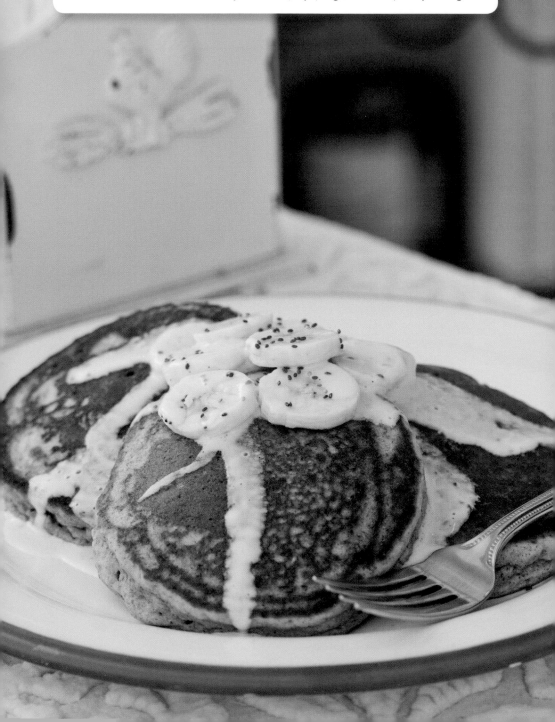

# Banana Chia Pancakes with Coconut Crème Sauce

*Chia seeds are loaded with omega-3s, fiber, and protein.
They are not just for Chia Pets anymore. It's easy to grind them up
in a coffee grinder or blender. These gluten-free pancakes are
sure to be a hit at your breakfast table any morning.*

Place the flour, chia seeds, baking soda, baking powder, and sea salt into a bowl and stir together. In a separate bowl, mash the peeled bananas into a paste or use a food processor. Add the mashed banana, agave nectar, coconut milk, cinnamon, and vanilla to the flour mixture and stir well to combine the batter. Heat a dollop of coconut oil on a nonstick skillet or griddle and pour the batter on it by ¼ cups. Let the pancakes cook until bubbly and the edges are somewhat dry, and then flip over and brown on the other side. If the batter thickens up too much, add a touch more coconut milk (this is the result of the chia seeds gelatinizing). Serve with Coconut Crème Sauce (recipe follows).

2 cups Bob's Red Mill Gluten-Free Flour

2 tablespoons chia seeds

1 teaspoon baking soda

1 teaspoon baking powder

½ teaspoon sea salt

2 ripe bananas

2 tablespoons agave nectar

1½ cups coconut milk

1 teaspoon cinnamon

1 teaspoon vanilla extract

1 tablespoon coconut oil for cooking pancakes

## Coconut Crème Sauce (1 cup)

¼ cup cashews, soaked for 2 hours

½ cup coconut milk (from a can)

3 Medjool dates, pitted

1 teaspoon vanilla extract

Pinch of sea salt

Place all of the ingredients in a blender, and blend until smooth

Per Serving: Calories 130, Total Fat 4g, Saturated Fat 2.5g, Cholesterol 0mg, Sodium 240mg, Carbohydrate 23g, Fiber 3g, Protein 2g
Coconut Crème Sauce: Calories 60, Total Fat 3.5g, Saturated Fat 2.5g, Cholesterol 0mg, Sodium 35mg, Carbohydrate 7g, Fiber 1g, Protein 1g

43

# Da Bomb Fruity Smoothie

*I love a fruit smoothie, and this one uses berries, kiwi, and banana. It's high in vitamin C and antioxidants! Use any kind of dairy-free milk you like.*

1¼ cups almond or coconut milk

1 ripe banana

1 ripe kiwi

Juice from ½ lime

½ cup frozen blueberries or pineapple

½ cup frozen strawberries

1 tablespoon agave nectar

Blend all of the ingredients together in a blender until smooth and creamy.

Per Serving: Calories 380, Total Fat 6g, Saturated Fat 0g, Cholesterol 0mg, Sodium 190mg, Carbohydrate 88g, Fiber 10g, Protein 4g

# Healer Ginger Tea

*I make this tea anytime I feel a slight cold coming on
or an imbalance in my body. It truly is healing, and it's also
great to sip after a meal for your digestion.*

Combine all of the ingredients except the honey in a small saucepan over medium heat. Bring to a simmer and let simmer for 5 to 7 minutes. Remove from the heat, add the honey to taste, and serve immediately.

2 cups water

1 tablespoon freshly grated ginger

Juice from ½ lemon

Dash cayenne pepper

Raw honey to taste

**CHEF'S TIP**

Fresh ginger is so good for your digestion. Peel your ginger first, and then use a microplane to grate the ginger into the water.

Per Serving: Calories 35, Total Fat 0g, Saturated Fat 0g, Cholesterol 0mg, Sodium 10mg, Carbohydrate 10g, Fiber 0g, Protein 0g

# Minty Hot Chocolate

*Hot chocolate on a cold winter's day is number one in my book.
This version is minty and delish.*

In a small saucepan over low heat, combine all of the ingredients and whisk well to combine. Be careful to not overheat and do not boil!

1½ cups unsweetened almond milk or coconut milk

1 tablespoon raw cacao powder

½ teaspoon vanilla extract

¼ teaspoon peppermint extract

2 teaspoons agave nectar (add more for more sweetness)

Per Serving: Calories 200, Total Fat 7g, Saturated Fat 2g, Cholesterol 0mg, Sodium 230mg, Carbohydrate 29g, Fiber 5g, Protein 5g

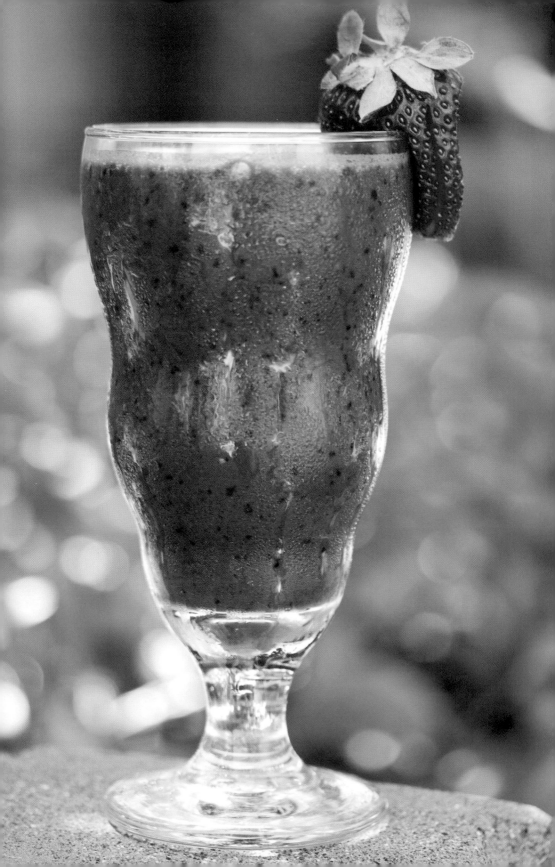

# Cherry Chocolate Smoothie

*Cherries and chocolate are my favorite combination in the world, so I had to blend them to make a delectable breakfast smoothie. This is also great to have as an afternoon revitalizer. Just add a scoop of protein powder and you'll be ready to take on the rest of the day.*

Blend all of the ingredients together in a blender until smooth and creamy.

½ cup coconut water

½ cup almond milk

1 cup of frozen organic cherries

1 small ripe banana, fresh or frozen

2 tablespoons raw cacao powder

1 teaspoon maca powder

1 tablespoon dark blue agave nectar or maple syrup

**Did You Know?** Maca is grown in central Peru and Bolivia at high altitudes. Since it has few natural pests, it is nearly always grown organically. Scientific studies of the plant, which Andeans have used for two thousand years, report that it may positively affect the endocrine system, promote energy, and aid sexual health in both men and women. Since it can cause gastric issues unless you cook it before eating, it's best to use the freeze-dried kind.

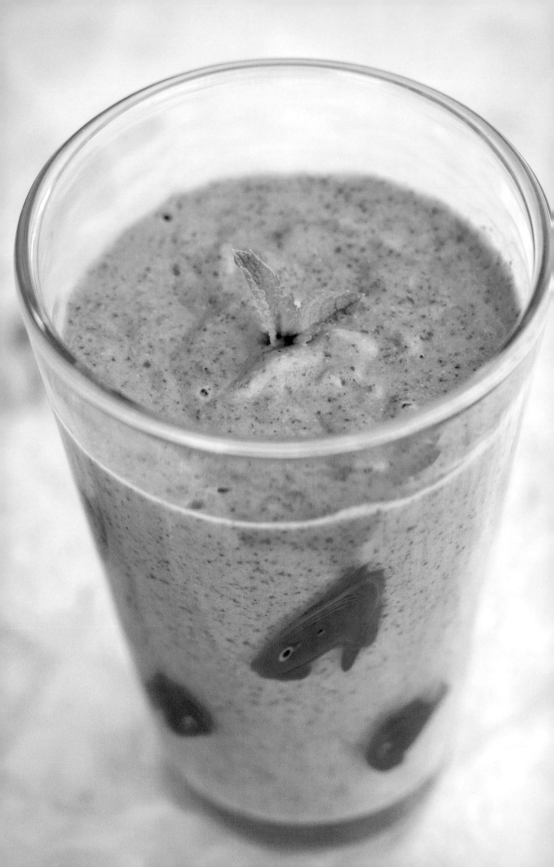

# Green Heaven
# Smoothie

*Get your greens in this deliciously thick and highly nutritious smoothie.*
*This is especially good for you first thing in the morning,*
*as it is alkalizing for the body. Ingesting alkaline foods regularly,*
*such as leafy greens, helps our body to fight disease.*
*Feel free to use any combination of greens you like.*

Blend all of the ingredients together in a blender until smooth and creamy. If your smoothie is too thick, add a dash more almond milk.

1 ripe banana, frozen

2 handfuls of spinach, kale, or romaine

1¼ cups almond milk

¼ avocado

1 tablespoon raw almond butter

1 tablespoon chia seeds

3 dates, pitted

Handful of ice

# Divine Coconutty Chai (Caffeine Free)

*I love chai; it's so warming and nourishing. This caffeine-free version is soothing to have in the evening before bed. The spices aid digestion and reduce inflammation.*

In a skillet over medium heat, toast the cardamom pods, cloves, and peppercorns until fragrant. Place the water on the stove in a pot and add the toasted pods, cloves, and peppercorns, along with the cinnamon sticks, ginger, and tea. Bring to a boil and then cover, reduce the heat, and simmer for approximately 7 minutes. Turn off the heat and let it steep for 15 minutes. Strain it through a fine mesh sieve, discarding the spices, then return the liquid to the pot and turn the heat to low. Add the coconut milk and maple syrup. Allow to heat through for approximately 1 minute. Do not boil.

12 whole green cardamom pods

12 whole cloves

20 black peppercorns

6 cups water

3 cinnamon sticks

6 slices gingerroot

2 tablespoons rooibos tea (loose)

2 cups canned coconut milk

2 tablespoons maple syrup

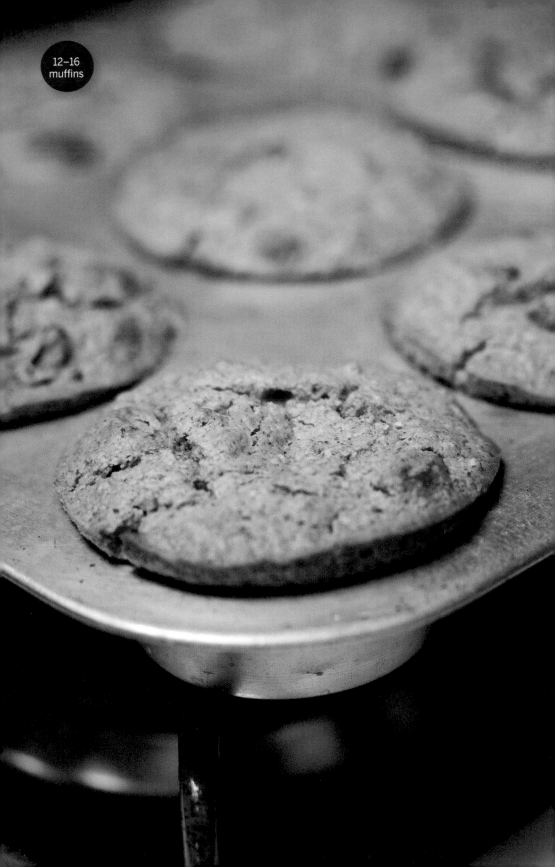

12–16
muffins

# Cherry Pecan Quinoa Muffins

*These muffins are flavorful and packed with protein.*
*The quinoa offers them a nutty flavor and a denser texture.*
*One of these babies will get you through*
*the morning and then some.*

Preheat the oven to 350 degrees F. Grease a muffin tin with coconut oil or cooking spray, or line with paper liners. Whisk the flour, baking powder, cinnamon, cloves, and nutmeg together in a large bowl and set aside. In a medium-size bowl, stir together the applesauce, agave nectar, cashew butter, coconut milk, vanilla, and sea salt. Fold the wet ingredients into the dry and stir using a wooden spoon to combine well. Fold in the quinoa, cherries, and pecans. Fill the muffin tins about two thirds full and bake for 20 minutes or until a toothpick inserted in the center comes out clean.

1 cup spelt or oat flour

1 tablespoon baking powder

1 teaspoon ground cinnamon

⅛ teaspoon cloves

¼ teaspoon ground nutmeg

2 tablespoons applesauce (no sugar added)

½ cup agave nectar or maple syrup

1 cup cashew or almond butter (smooth, not chunky)

⅔ cup coconut milk

2 teaspoons vanilla extract

¼ teaspoon sea salt

⅔ cup cooked and cooled quinoa

½ cup chopped dried cherries

½ cup roughly chopped pecans

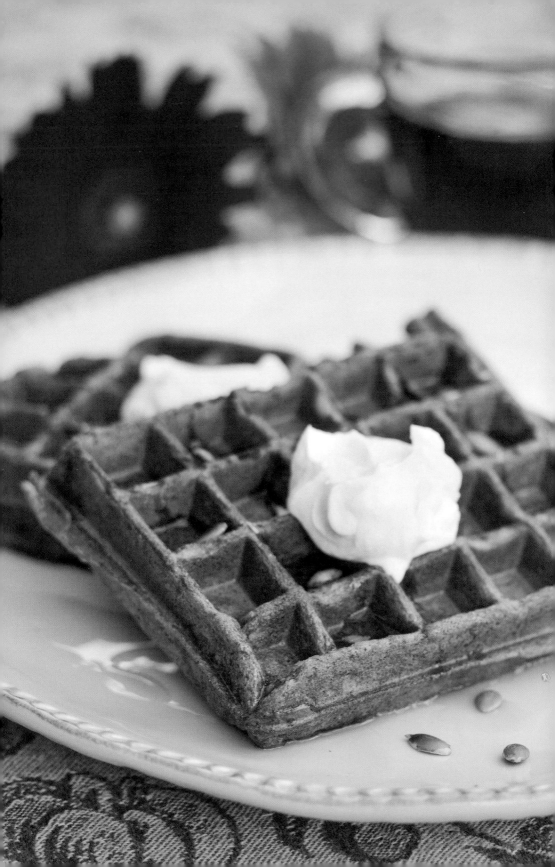

# Pumpkin Pie Waffles

6 six-inch waffles

*These are an awesome weekend treat to have with the family, especially at holiday time. Warming scents of cloves, ginger, and cinnamon will permeate your home with cozy goodness— a perfect and healthy winter comfort food.*

In a small bowl, combine the almond milk with the apple cider vinegar and set aside to "curdle." Mix the baking flour, xanthan gum, pumpkin pie spice, cloves, cinnamon, baking powder, baking soda, and salt in a large bowl using a fork. In a separate medium-size bowl, combine the milk mixture, pumpkin, agave nectar, applesauce, and flaxseed eggs. Add the wet mixture to the dry ingredients and mix well with a fork. Pour the batter onto a preheated, greased waffle iron and cook until brown and crispy.

1½ cups almond or rice milk

2 teaspoons apple cider vinegar

2¼ cups Bob's Red Mill All Purpose Gluten-Free Baking Flour

1 teaspoon xanthan gum

2 teaspoons pumpkin pie spice

¼ teaspoon cloves

1 teaspoon cinnamon

1 teaspoon baking powder

1 teaspoon baking soda

½ teaspoon sea salt

1 cup canned pumpkin

3 tablespoons agave nectar

3 tablespoons cinnamon applesauce

2 flaxseed eggs (see "How to Make Flaxseed Eggs" on page 26)

One 9-inch loaf

# Gluten-Free Zucchini Bread

*This light yet nutritionally dense bread is great in the morning or as an afternoon snack. Zucchini is high in potassium, which is calming to the system. No reason to feel guilty having a slice or two with these great benefits!*

2 cups Bob's Red Mill All Purpose Gluten-Free Baking Flour

½ cup ground flaxseed or chia seeds

2 teaspoons baking powder

2 teaspoons baking soda

1 teaspoon sea salt

2 teaspoons ground cinnamon

2 teaspoons ground ginger

½ cup melted coconut oil or avocado oil

¾ cup maple syrup

¾ cup almond or coconut milk

2 teaspoons vanilla extract

2 cups shredded zucchini

⅓ cup chopped walnuts

Preheat the oven to 350 degrees F. Lightly grease a loaf pan with nonstick spray or coconut oil. In a medium-size bowl, combine baking flour, flaxseed, baking powder, baking soda, salt, cinnamon, and ginger using a fork. Add coconut oil, maple syrup, milk, and vanilla and stir until smooth. Gently fold in the zucchini and walnuts and combine until evenly distributed throughout the batter. Pour the batter into the loaf pan and bake in the center of the oven for about 45 minutes. Bread will be done when a toothpick inserted into the center comes out clean. Remove from the oven and cool on a wire rack for about 15 minutes. Remove from the pan and slice.

Per Serving: Calories 280, Total Fat 17g, Saturated Fat 11g, Cholesterol 0mg, Sodium 480mg, Carbohydrate 32g, Fiber 4g, Protein 4g

# Chapter 2

# *Nosh, Nibble, and Dip Away*

**W**ho doesn't love to do all of these? This chapter is loaded with party foods—foods that are fun to take to picnics, campouts, potlucks, and any other kind of party. These celebratory foods are finger-licking, lip-smackingly good and will tickle your tummy with flavors galore. So snack, nosh, and nibble away!

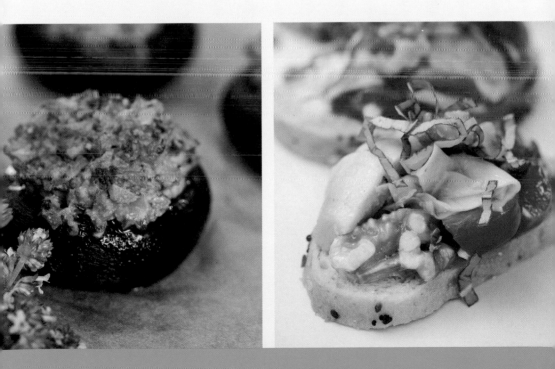

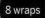

# Thai-Style Tempeh Lettuce Wraps

*Lettuce wraps are fun, flavorful, and simple to make.
Not only are they great for parties, they are also a great afternoon
snack instead of a candy bar or some other sugary food that will put you
into a midday coma. Whip the filling up the night before and tote them
to work with you for a crunchy, healthy, and satisfying snack.*

In a large skillet, heat the sesame oil over medium heat and sauté the garlic and ginger for about 2 minutes. Add the bell pepper and carrots and sauté until soft. Add the crumbled tempeh and sauté for about 5 minutes, stirring well to combine, until it is lightly browned.

In a blender combine the chili paste, miso, sesame oil, agave nectar, Braggs, and water. Blend until smooth. Add this to the tempeh mixture and stir to combine. Let it heat through for about 3 to 5 minutes.

*To assemble:* Scoop about a ¼ cup of the tempeh mixture onto a lettuce leaf and top with cucumber and bean sprouts. Sprinkle with sesame seeds and cilantro, if using, and roll and enjoy.

1 tablespoon sesame oil

2 teaspoons fresh minced garlic

2 teaspoons peeled and grated ginger

½ red bell pepper, deseeded and cut into long, thin strips

1 carrot, peeled and cut into matchsticks

2 8-ounce packages tempeh, crumbled into a bowl

2 tablespoons red chili paste

1 tablespoon mellow white miso paste

1 tablespoon toasted sesame oil

1 tablespoon agave nectar

1 tablespoon Braggs Aminos or low-sodium tamari

¼ cup water

8 butter lettuce or Bibb lettuce leaves, washed and dried

½ cucumber, peeled and cut into thin, long strips

½ cup mung bean sprouts or any sprouts

Sesame seeds, for garnish (optional)

Chopped cilantro for garnish (optional)

# Stuffed Mushroom Poppers

6–8 servings

Preheat the oven to 350 degrees F and lightly grease a baking pan.

Wash the mushrooms well. Pull the stems off of the mushrooms, chop, and set aside. Heat the oil in a large pan over medium heat, add the diced onion, and sauté until translucent. Add the garlic, mushroom stems, thyme, parsley, and basil. Stir to combine and cook down until the stems are soft. Deglaze the pan with vinegar and then add the water. Add the chopped spinach and let the mixture cook about 2 to 3 minutes longer until the liquid is almost evaporated. Remove the pan from the heat and set aside.

Grind the walnuts in a coffee grinder, blender, or food processor. Put the walnuts into a small bowl and mix in the salt, pepper, and nutritional yeast. Stir into the pan with the mushroom and spinach mixture until well combined. Fill the mushroom caps with the filling.

Place the mushroom caps in a single layer on the baking pan and bake for 15 to 20 minutes. The mushrooms will turn golden, and the stuffing should begin to brown.

- 12–16 large stuffing mushrooms
- 2 tablespoons extra virgin olive oil
- 1 medium red onion, diced
- 2 garlic cloves, minced
- 1 tablespoon fresh chopped thyme
- 2 tablespoons fresh chopped parsley
- 1 tablespoon fresh chopped basil
- 2 tablespoons champagne or sherry vinegar
- 2 tablespoons water
- 1 bunch fresh spinach leaves, chopped
- ½ cup toasted walnuts
- ½ teaspoon sea salt
- ¼ teaspoon freshly ground pepper
- 1 tablespoon nutritional yeast

Per Serving: Calories 110, Total Fat 8g, Saturated Fat 1g, Cholesterol 0mg, Sodium 190mg, Carbohydrate 6g, Fiber 2g, Protein 5g

61

# Veggie Seed Roll-Ups

*I love to gather together a few of my friends and
have a roll-up party. I usually make the "pâté" the day prior,
so the flavors really have a chance to meld. Remember, these
don't need to look perfect to impress because they will
taste so great—and I promise they will!*

Lay 1 nori sheet, rough side up, on a cutting board. Spread a thin layer (about 3 tablespoons) of Sunflower Seed Pâté evenly on the nori sheet. Stack the carrot strip, cucumber strip, avocado slice, and sprouts in a narrow line 1 inch from the long edge of the nori sheet. Fold the nori sheet over the vegetables and roll the sheet away from you as tightly as possible. Dab the edge of the nori sheet with water to seal and close. Repeat with the remaining ingredients. Place in the refrigerator for about 20 minutes to firm up. With a serrated knife, cut each roll into bite-size pieces and serve.

8 sheets nori (thin sheets of dried seaweed)

½ cup Sunflower Seed Pâté (page 77)

2 carrots, peeled and cut into long, thin strips

1 cucumber, peeled, deseeded, and cut into thin strips

1 avocado, halved and thinly sliced

1 8-ounce container daikon sprouts or sunflower sprouts

Per Serving: Calories 130, Total Fat 11g, Saturated Fat 3g, Cholesterol 10mg, Sodium 85mg, Carbohydrate 6g, Fiber 2g, Protein 5g

63

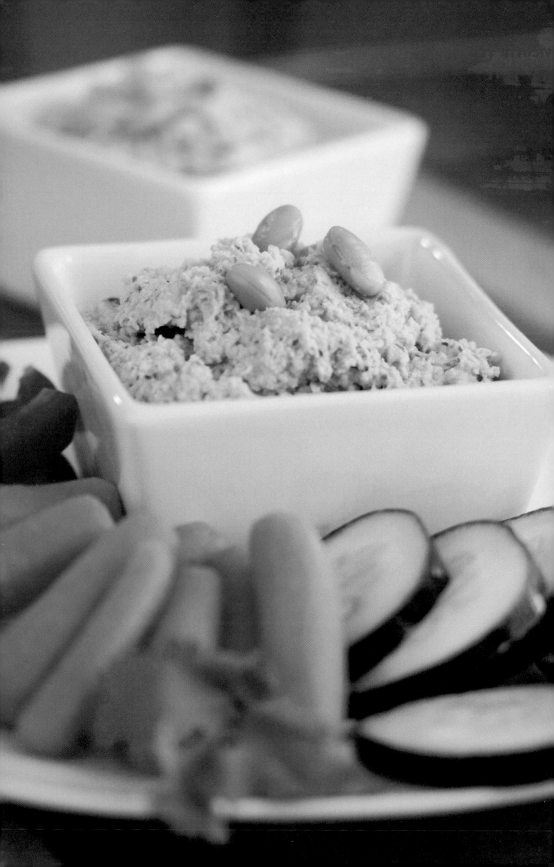

# Kickin' Edamame Dip

*Edamame, also known as soybean, is high in fiber and protein. It's easily found in your grocer's freezer, but make sure you buy preshelled edamame for ease. I also recommend buying organic, as oftentimes nonorganic contains genetically modified organisms (GMOs).*

Put all of the ingredients into a food processor except for the olive oil and lime juice. Puree until combined. Add the olive oil and lime juice and puree more, scraping the sides of the processor bowl frequently. If you like a smoother consistency, add purified water 1 tablespoon at a time while the processor is running, until the desired texture is achieved.

1 package (16 ounces) frozen and shelled edamame, cooked according to instructions

4 large garlic cloves, chopped

1¼ teaspoons sea salt

½ teaspoon ground coriander

1 teaspoon ground cumin

¼ teaspoon cayenne

¼ cup fresh cilantro

4–6 tablespoons extra virgin olive oil

¼ cup freshly squeezed lime juice

Per Serving: Calories 70, Total Fat 6g, Saturated Fat 0.5g, Cholesterol 0mg, Sodium 230mg, Carbohydrate 3g, Fiber 1g, Protein 2g

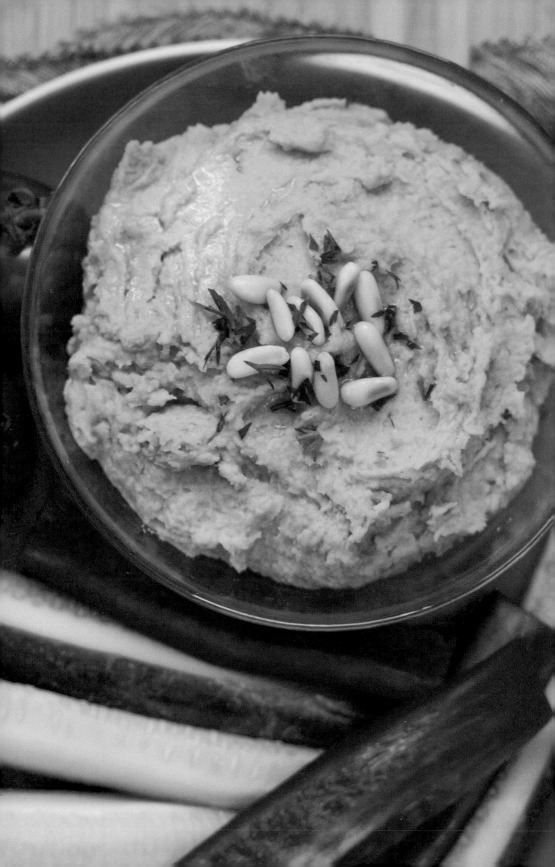

# Garnet Hummus

**About 2 cups**

*I love this sweet twist on classic hummus.
It's always a favorite at parties and is usually the first dip
to be wiped clean. You might want to make two batches,
as it is quite addicting! Serve it alongside a huge tray
of fresh veggies and some gluten-free crackers.*

Preheat the oven to 400 degrees F. Poke holes in the yams with a fork. Place the yams on a baking sheet lined with parchment paper. Bake for approximately 40 minutes or until soft. Remove from the oven and allow to cool. Once cool, remove the skin and scoop the flesh out into a food processor bowl.

Add the remaining ingredients to the food processor bowl except for the olive oil. Puree until well combined, adding the olive oil while blending. Blend until smooth and creamy, adding more oil if needed or a small amount of water if the hummus is too thick. Be sure to scrape down the sides of the bowl a few times to incorporate all of the ingredients.

1 pound garnet yams, washed well, skin left on

Juice from 1 large lemon

1 teaspoon cumin powder

1 teaspoon sea salt

Dash cayenne pepper (use more if you like spice)

1 tablespoon agave nectar

1 15-ounce can chickpeas or garbanzo beans, drained and rinsed well

2 tablespoons tahini

3 tablespoons extra virgin olive oil (more if necessary)

Per Serving: Calories 50, Total Fat 2g, Saturated Fat 0g, Cholesterol 0mg, Sodium 75mg, Carbohydrate 6g, Fiber 1g, Protein 1g

67

# Green Earth Dip

*This dip is green (both in color and in Earth friendliness), creamy, and dreamy. Using cashews as a base, it's got a bit of a sweet and savory flavor all in one bite. Add any type of fresh herbs you want. I love the combination of cilantro and parsley together, but feel free to use a dill and basil combination if you don't like the others.*

Puree all of the ingredients in a food processor except for the olive oil. While the processor is still running, pour the olive oil into the processor. Add water 1 tablespoon at a time if you want a creamier consistency. Process until smooth. Be sure to scrape the sides of the processor bowl frequently to ensure that all of the ingredients are well blended.

1½ cups cashews, soaked in water for 2 hours or more

3 scallions, chopped

1 garlic clove

3 tablespoons fresh cilantro

3 tablespoons fresh parsley

1 tablespoon honey mustard

1 tablespoon brown rice vinegar

2 teaspoons white mellow miso

2 teaspoons agave nectar

½ teaspoon sea salt

Juice from 1 lemon or lime

3 tablespoons olive oil

Water, as needed

Per Serving: Calories 90, Total Fat 7g, Saturated Fat 1g, Cholesterol 0mg, Sodium 65mg, Carbohydrate 5g, Fiber 1g, Protein 2g

69

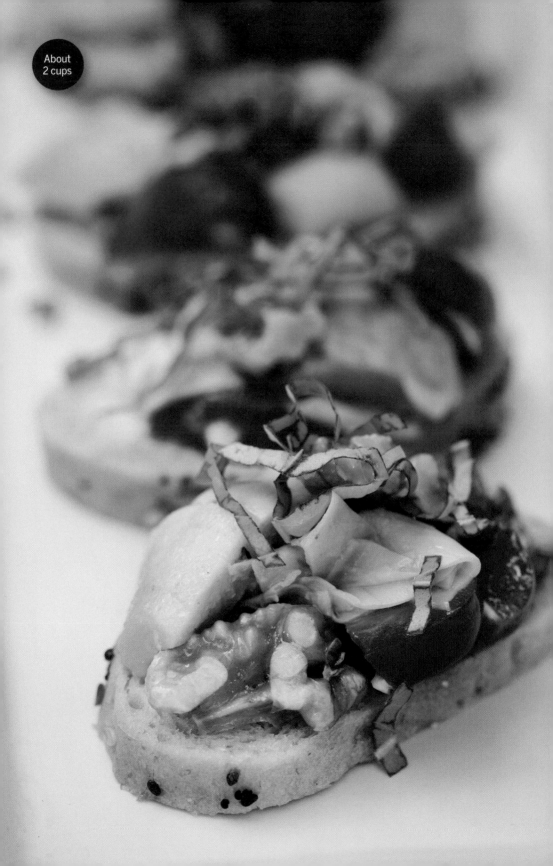

# Heart-Full Bruschetta

*Bruschetta was a staple in my Italian household growing up.*
*I added some artichoke hearts to this version for a little more texture*
*and flavor. Serve this on top of gluten-free crackers or*
*warm, crusty sourdough bread. It's delicious!*

Place the tomatoes, artichoke hearts, garlic, and walnuts in a medium-size bowl. Add the lemon zest and juice, vinegar, basil, and olive oil. Season with salt and pepper.

4 ripe plum tomatoes, coarsely chopped

1 cup frozen artichoke hearts, thawed and coarsely chopped (you can also substitute 1 cup or 8 ounces of canned artichokes)

1–2 cloves garlic, minced (depending on personal preference)

¼ cup toasted and chopped walnuts

Zest and juice from 1 lemon

2 tablespoons rice vinegar

5–8 large fresh basil leaves, chopped

3 tablespoons extra virgin olive oil

Salt and freshly ground black pepper, to taste

Per Serving: Calories 35, Total Fat 3.5g, Saturated Fat 0g, Cholesterol 0mg, Sodium 5mg, Carbohydrate 2g, Fiber 1g, Protein 1g

71

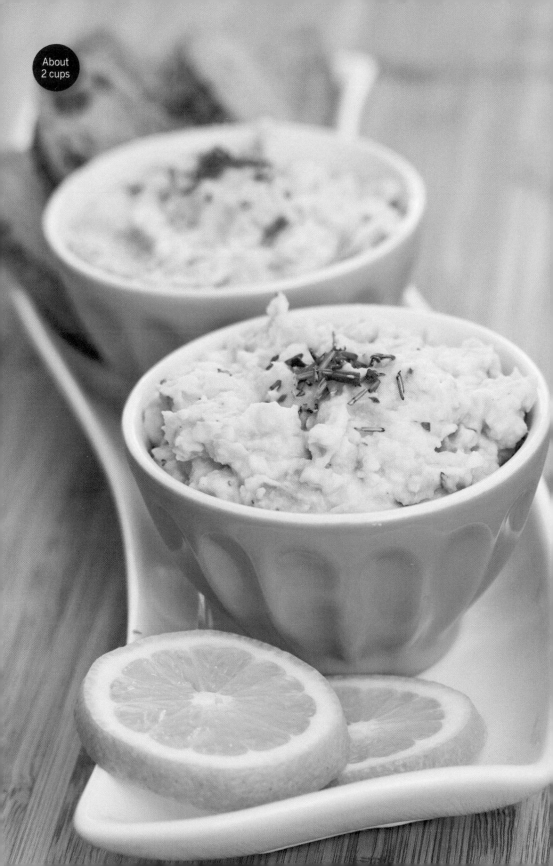

# Artichoke and White Bean Dip
# with Rosemary

*Artichoke hearts and white beans make for a crunky
(that's creamy and chunky) dip that is loaded with flavor and great to
serve at any party. I love to spread this on a gluten-free or sprouted grain
tortilla topped with fresh veggies and then roll it up for a snack.*

In a skillet over low heat, heat the olive oil and sauté the garlic and shallot until soft. Put the garlic and shallot mixture into a food processor, along with the remaining ingredients, except for the artichoke hearts. Process until smooth. Add the artichokes and pulse, but you still want some chunks to remain intact. Season with salt and pepper.

2 teaspoons extra virgin olive oil

2 garlic cloves, peeled and minced

1 shallot, peeled and finely chopped

2 tablespoons fresh-squeezed
   lemon juice

¼ cup grapeseed Vegenaise

1 tablespoon apple cider vinegar

2 cups canned white beans,
   drained and rinsed

¼ teaspoon salt

½ teaspoon chopped fresh rosemary

½ teaspoon powdered mustard

¼ teaspoon pepper

1½ cups frozen artichoke hearts,
   thawed (jarred or canned are fine,
   too, but drain first)

Sea salt and ground pepper, to taste

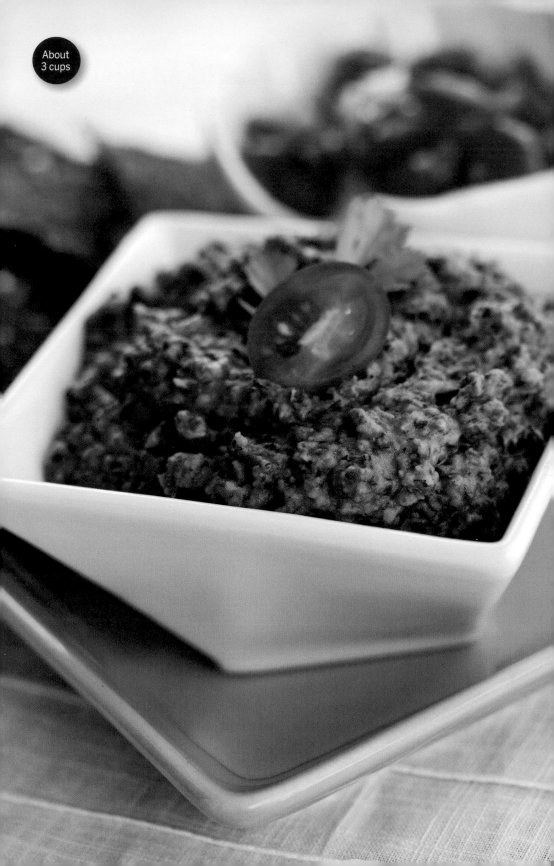

# Arriba Black Bean Dip

*This dip is smoky, spicy, and just plain great!*
*Serve it with some baked blue corn chips or cut-up veggies.*
*It will transport you right to the sandy beaches of Mexico!*

Heat 1 tablespoon of the olive oil in a skillet over medium heat and sauté the jalapeño, red bell pepper, onion, and garlic until soft. Add the cumin and chili powder and stir while cooking to incorporate. Remove from heat when all of the ingredients are soft and somewhat caramelized.

In a food processor, place the pepper mixture, black beans, apple cider vinegar, honey, and salt. Puree all of the ingredients while pouring the remaining 2 tablespoons of olive oil into the processor while running. Make sure you remove the lid and scrape the sides and puree again. Serve warm or chilled.

3 tablespoons olive oil

½ jalapeño pepper, deseeded and minced

1 red bell pepper, deseeded and diced

1 small red onion, finely diced

1 clove garlic, minced

1 teaspoon cumin

¼ teaspoon chipotle chili powder

1½ cups canned black beans, rinsed

1 tablespoon apple cider vinegar

2 teaspoons honey or maple syrup

½ teaspoon sea salt

Per Serving: Calories 45, Total Fat 2.5g, Saturated Fat 0g, Cholesterol 0mg, Sodium 65mg, Carbohydrate 5g, Fiber 1g, Protein 1g

75

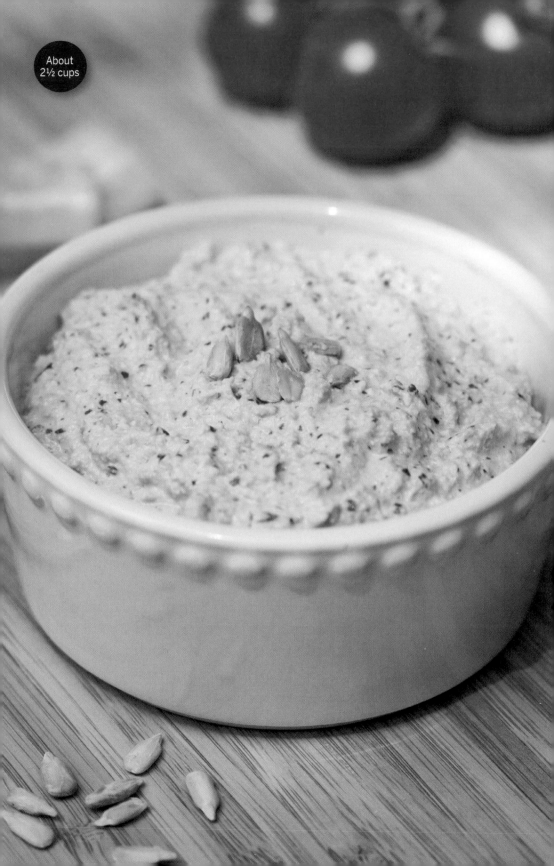

About
2½ cups

# Sunflower Seed "Pâté"

*I love this veganized version of pâté because it's
healthy, tasty, and a hit on any party table. Make sure to soak
the sunflower seeds for the allotted time so that the consistency is
creamy. This is great served with raw veggies on the side.*

Drain the water from the sunflower seeds. Place all of the ingredients except for the olive oil in a food processor and puree. While the food processor is still running, add the olive oil until creamy and smooth (add more or less depending on the consistency you desire). If you want an even creamier consistency, add a small amount of water while the processor is running.

2 cups shelled sunflower seeds, soaked in water for 4 hours

1 yellow bell pepper, deseeded and chopped

1 large handful fresh parsley

1 large handful fresh basil

1 tablespoon apple cider vinegar

2 tablespoons lemon juice

1 clove garlic

1 tablespoon Braggs Aminos or low-sodium tamari

2–4 tablespoons extra virgin olive oil

**Karmic Health Tip:** *All pâtés are made from duck livers, which tend to be fatty and not so healthy for you. This version has a similar consistency but with a great taste and health benefits to boot.*

Per Serving: Calories 90, Total Fat 8g, Saturated Fat 1g, Cholesterol 0mg, Sodium 30mg, Carbohydrate 3g, Fiber 1g, Protein 3g

77

# Spicy Olive Tapenade

*Tapenade is my favorite served on crackers with
a little dash of hummus plopped right on top. Olives are high
in healthy fats and great for your skin, hair, and nails.
You can use any combination of olives. I've used my
two favorites, but feel free to get creative!*

1 cup pitted kalamata olives
(Greek-style olives)

1 cup pitted green olives

1 large roasted red pepper,
deseeded and chopped
(you can also substitute
1 large whole roasted
pepper from a jar)

¼ teaspoon red pepper flakes

3 garlic cloves

3 tablespoons olive oil

In a food processor bowl, combine all of the ingredients except the olive oil. Puree, and while the motor is running, drizzle the olive oil in the top until well combined and smooth. Make sure to scrape down the side of the processor bowl and reprocess.

Chef's tip: Roasting peppers is simple and easy. Wash and dry them, throw them on a parchment-lined baking sheet, and coat with a light mist of olive oil spray. Bake in the oven at 400 degrees F for 15 to 20 minutes or until the skin is brown and blistery. Remove from the oven, let cool, and then peel skin and deseed.

Per Serving: Calories 70, Total Fat 6g, Saturated Fat 0.5g, Cholesterol 0mg, Sodium 250mg, Carbohydrate 2g, Fiber 0g, Protein 0g

# Cheezy Popcorn

3 servings

In a large pot with a fitted lid, heat the coconut oil over medium heat until melted. Add the popcorn kernels and place a lid on the pot. Wait until the first kernel pops and then lower the heat a tad. The popcorn will continue to pop; you do not need to shake the pot, but you can if you like. Cook until you hear the popping slow (when you hear a few seconds between the popping), as you don't want it to burn. Remove the lid and pour the popcorn into a large bowl. Season with salt, pepper, and nutritional yeast flakes to taste for a "cheesy" flavor. Mix well or shake in a bag!

- 1 tablespoon extra virgin coconut oil
- ½ cup organic popcorn kernels (it's best to buy in bulk to save money)
- Sea salt and pepper, to taste
- 1–2 tablespoons nutritional yeast flakes, or more to taste

**Kettle corn variation:** For kettle corn, leave out the nutritional yeast and drizzle 1–2 tablespoons of agave nectar over the popcorn. Stir to combine and salt to taste.

Per Serving: Calories 170, Total Fat 6g, Saturated Fat 0.5g, Cholesterol 0mg, Sodium 0mg, Carbohydrate 23g, Fiber 6g, Protein 5g

79

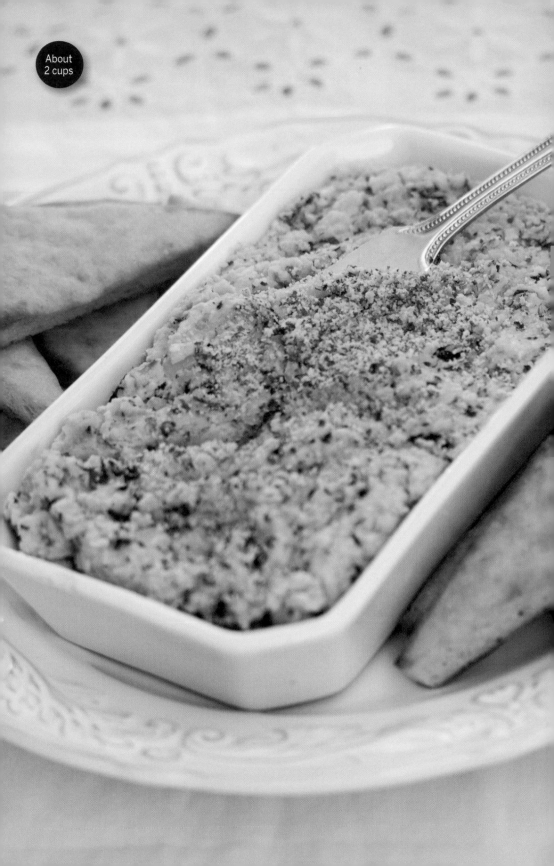

# Creamy Spinach Artichoke Dip

Preheat the oven to 400 degrees F. Drain the cashews. In a food processor or blender, blend the cashews and beans with the water, lemon juice, Vegenaise, and nutritional yeast until creamy. If mixture is too thick, add water 1 tablespoon at a time until thick and creamy. Scrape into a bowl and set aside.

Heat the olive oil in a skillet over medium heat and sauté the onion and garlic until soft. Add the artichokes and sauté until lightly browned. Add the spinach and let it wilt down, about 2 to 3 minutes. Pour into a large bowl and add the cashew and bean mixture, salt, and red pepper flakes (to taste). Stir to combine well. Pour into a lightly oiled casserole dish and top with bread crumbs. Cover with foil and bake for about 15 minutes. Remove foil and bake 10 minutes more until a little browned.

½ cup cashews, soaked for 20 minutes

1 15-ounce can cannellini (white) beans, drained and rinsed

½ cup water

2 tablespoons lemon juice

¼ cup grapeseed Vegenaise

3 tablespoons nutritional yeast

1 tablespoon extra virgin olive oil

1 medium yellow onion, diced

4 garlic cloves, minced

1½ cups thawed and chopped frozen artichoke hearts (or substitute 1½ cups jarred artichoke hearts)

3 cups chopped fresh spinach (chopped small)

1 teaspoon sea salt

dash red pepper flakes

¼ cup gluten-free bread crumbs

Per Serving: Calories 35, Total Fat 2g, Saturated Fat 0g, Cholesterol 0mg, Sodium 80mg, Carbohydrate 4g, Fiber 1g, Protein 2g

81

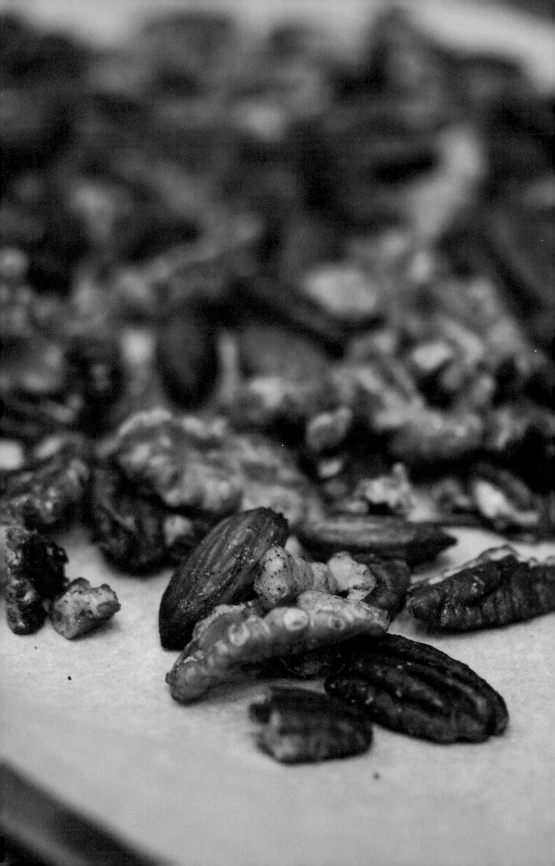

# Roasted and Spiced Mixed Nuts

2 cups

*These roasted beauties are a hit on any appetizer table.
I love to throw them on a salad or just keep a bowlful on my
buffet table for people to snack on anytime.*

Preheat the oven to 375 degrees F. In a medium saucepan over low heat, combine all of the ingredients except the nuts. Heat through, stirring frequently, until well combined. Add the nuts and toss to combine. Spread the nuts onto a large rimmed baking sheet lined with parchment paper and bake until golden and fragrant, about 12 to 15 minutes, stirring about halfway through. (Nuts can burn very quickly, so keep an eye on them.) Put the pan on a cooling rack and let the nuts cool.

2 tablespoons extra virgin olive oil or coconut oil

2 tablespoons chopped fresh rosemary

2 tablespoons agave nectar or maple syrup

½ teaspoon cayenne pepper

¼ teaspoon cinnamon

1 tablespoon coarse sea salt

¼ pound raw, shelled walnuts

¼ pound raw, shelled pecans

¼ pound raw, shelled pistachios

¼ pound raw, shelled almonds

# Peanut Sauce

*This is great to use as a dip, salad dressing, or
a sauce for your favorite Thai dish. It's simple to make
and loaded with healthy fats and protein!*

1 cup coconut milk

3 tablespoons chunky peanut
butter

2 tablespoons Braggs Aminos
or low-sodium tamari

¼ teaspoon red pepper flakes

2 tablespoons rice wine vinegar

2 teaspoons maple syrup

1 teaspoon arrowroot powder

Combine all of the ingredients in a
blender and blend until smooth.

Per Serving: Calories 60, Total Fat 6g, Saturated Fat 3.5g, Cholesterol 0mg, Sodium 110mg, Carbohydrate 2g, Fiber 0g, Protein 1g

# Chipotle Cashew Cheeze Sauce

*Café Gratitude, a popular vegan restaurant in
Southern California, whips up this cashew-based "cheese,"
so I had to create my own version! It's smoky and creamy, and it's
really good heated and poured over Blissed-Out Herb-Roasted
Taters (page 185) or as a topping on nachos, or a sauce
for Mac and Ch-ch-cheeeeze (page 147).*

Drain the water from the cashews. Place all the ingredients in a blender cup with just enough water to barely cover. Blend until very smooth. Add more water if the mixture is too thick or if you're having trouble blending the ingredients. This mixture should be a fairly thick sauce.

2 cups cashews, soaked in water for 4 hours

¼ cup nutritional yeast flakes

1 tablespoon lemon juice

½ teaspoon chipotle chili powder

½ teaspoon garlic powder

½ teaspoon sea salt

¼ teaspoon smoked paprika (optional)

Filtered water

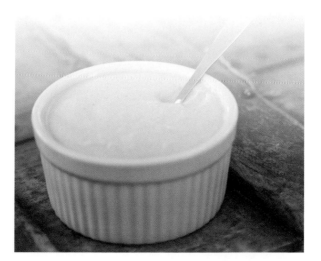

Per Serving: Calories 70, Total Fat 5g, Saturated Fat 1g, Cholesterol 0mg, Sodium 120mg, Carbohydrate 5g, Fiber 1g, Protein 4g

85

**Serves 2**

# Sweet and Savory Kale "Chips"

*This is one of my favorite ways to eat kale. I always make two batches before I go on the road and take them with me. They are so much better than chips for a snack. They're a bit savory and a bit sweet—I think they will turn you into a kale chip convert!*

1 large head dino kale
  (looks like dinosaur skin)

Juice of 1 lemon

2 tablespoons olive oil

2 tablespoons creamy almond
  butter

1 tablespoon agave nectar or
  maple syrup

1 tablespoon nutritional yeast

½ teaspoon sea salt

Preheat the oven to 300 degrees F. Strip the stems from the dino kale and wash well. Place in a large bowl. Blend or whisk the remaining ingredients together until smooth, then pour over the kale. Toss with your hands to coat each leaf. Place the kale in a single layer onto nonstick cookie sheets (or line regular cookie sheets with parchment paper). Bake for 10 to 15 minutes, until edges are crispy. Be careful not to burn. Also, keep in mind that the kale will only get crispy around the edges, not crispy all the way through. Enjoy these within one day, as they will lose their crispness if stored longer than that.

Per Serving: Calories 380, Total Fat 24g, Saturated Fat 3g, Cholesterol 0mg, Sodium 720mg, Carbohydrate 35g, Fiber 7g, Protein 13g

# Charlie's Tomato Sauce
# Marinara

*This is the California-ized version of the tomato sauce my Italian father used to make when I was a kid. I kept it simple and left out the blanching and hand-peeling of the tomatoes to save you some time in the kitchen. The flavor is delish and just a bit zestier than Dad's due to my secret ingredient: balsamic vinegar. Prego!*

In a large stockpot, heat the olive oil over medium heat and sauté the onion, garlic, and mushrooms until soft and caramelized, about 5 to 7 minutes. Add the thyme, red pepper flakes, and oregano, and stir to incorporate and release the fragrance and flavor of the herbs. Add the crushed tomatoes and tomato paste. Reduce the heat and simmer 20 to 30 minutes. Add the tamari, agave nectar, and balsamic vinegar, and stir well. Simmer 5 to 10 minutes more. Season with salt and pepper, and top with fresh basil. This stores well in the refrigerator for at least five days (and it freezes well, too). Simply reheat the defrosted marinara sauce in a sauce pan over low heat.

2 tablespoons extra virgin olive oil

1 medium red onion, diced

4 cloves garlic, minced

1 cup sliced shiitake mushrooms (stems removed)

1 teaspoon dried thyme

¼ teaspoon red pepper flakes

2 teaspoons dried oregano

2 28-ounce cans fire-roasted crushed tomatoes

3 ounces tomato paste

1 tablespoon tamari

2 teaspoons agave nectar

1 tablespoon balsamic vinegar

Sea salt and freshly ground black pepper, to taste

2 tablespoons finely chopped fresh basil

# Savory Golden Mushroom Gravy

*Finally, a vegan gravy that's worthy to be on the table with other holiday fare. I love to make my famous Chickpea Fillets (page 149) and top them with this scrumptious golden gravy or even scoop it on top of some mashed red bliss potatoes!*

½ cup nutritional yeast flakes

½ cup brown rice flour

3 tablespoons extra virgin olive oil

½ cup diced sweet yellow onion

2 cloves garlic, minced

2 cups finely chopped wild mushrooms (I like a mixture of portobello, shiitake, or oyster)

1½ teaspoons dried sage

1½ teaspoons dried thyme

1½ teaspoons dried tarragon

2 cups vegetable broth

¼ cup low-sodium tamari or Braggs Aminos

½ cup unsweetened almond or coconut milk (I like So Delicious brand)

½ teaspoon ground black pepper

In a small bowl, whisk together the nutritional yeast flakes and rice flour. Set aside.

Heat the olive oil in a large saucepan over medium heat. Sauté the onion, garlic, and mushrooms until softened, about 10 minutes. Add the sage, thyme, and tarragon, and stir to release the flavors of the herbs. Whisk in the flour mixture thoroughly to combine and then whisk in the vegetable broth, tamari, almond milk, and ground black pepper. Keep stirring frequently until the gravy is thick and creamy. Serve immediately.

Per Serving: Calories 130, Total Fat 6g, Saturated Fat 1g, Cholesterol 0mg, Sodium 440mg, Carbohydrate 14g, Fiber 3g, Protein 6g

# Chile Ranchero Sauce

*This Chile Ranchero Sauce is awesome to put on tacos or to use when making the Cha-Cha Enchiladarole (page 164). You are welcome to use poblano chilies if you want it a bit spicier. Roasting these peppers and peeling them is part of the fun! If you are in a hurry, you can buy chilies in a can and use them instead, but fresh is always best!*

Preheat the oven to 400 degrees F. Roast the chilies in the oven for about 20 to 25 minutes or until brown and blistery. Remove from the oven and let cool. Once cool, peel the skin, deseed, and chop roughly. Set aside.

Heat the olive oil in a saucepan over medium-low heat and sauté the onion and garlic until soft. Add the chili powder, cumin, and oregano. Stir well to combine and release the flavors of the spices and herbs. Add the tomatoes and chili peppers. Turn the heat to low and simmer for 15 to 20 minutes, uncovered. Add the agave nectar and salt and cook about 2 minutes longer. Remove from the heat and with a hand blender or regular blender, puree until smooth.

2 Anaheim chili peppers, roasted, peeled, deseeded, and roughly chopped

2 tablespoons extra virgin olive oil

1 medium sweet yellow onion, finely diced

2 cloves garlic, minced

2 teaspoons dried chili powder

1 teaspoon ground cumin

1 teaspoon Mexican oregano or marjoram

1 28-ounce can fire-roasted diced tomatoes with juice

1 teaspoon agave nectar

1½ teaspoons sea salt

Per Serving: Calories 15, Total Fat 1g, Saturated Fat 0g, Cholesterol 0mg, Sodium 150mg, Carbohydrate 2g, Fiber 0g, Protein 0g

89

# Dreamy Avocado "Mayo"

*It's not really mayo, but it could take its place
without anyone complaining. Use this as a spread on
sandwiches or as a dip for your favorite raw veggies.
It's loaded with healthy fats and flavor.*

2 ripe avocados, skins removed

1 garlic clove, finely minced

2 teaspoons maple syrup or
  agave nectar

2 tablespoons apple cider
  vinegar

Juice of one lime or lemon

¼ teaspoon sea salt

¼ cup olive oil

2 tablespoons water

In a blender, combine all of the ingredients together and blend until smooth and creamy. Store in a tightly covered container for two days.

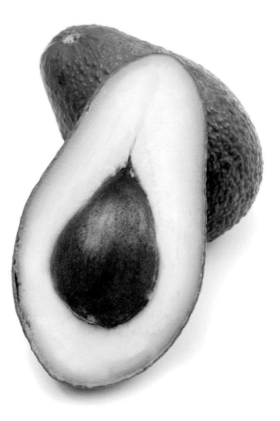

Per Serving: Calories 180, Total Fat 17g, Saturated Fat 2g, Cholesterol 0mg, Sodium 100mg, Carbohydrate 8g, Fiber 2g, Protein 2g

**Chapter 3**

# *Hearty One-Pot Soups and Stews*

*T*his chapter is one of my favorite parts of the book, because almost all of these dishes can be made in one pot! I love to make a few different soups on a weekend and freeze them for future noshing. Most of these recipes can also be made within an hour or less from start to finish, so they are perfect to throw on the stove and then go relax with your family or friends. They're hearty, satisfying, and super tasty!

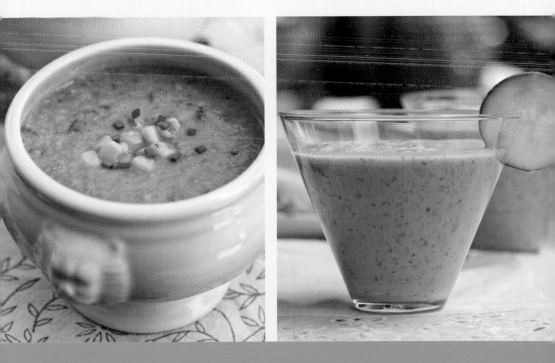

**Did You Know?** Most soups start with a base of carrot, onion, and celery. It's known as *mirepoix* in France. I love to add garlic to this trio for a little extra punch and antiviral properties to boot!

# Lentil Soup

*I love this soup because it's nutritious and perfectly warming on a cold, wintry day! It's almost a meal on its own, as it packs tons of protein and fiber. Serve with a leafy green salad and you'll make the perfect lunch or dinner combination.*

Heat the oil in a large soup pot over medium heat. Add the onion, garlic, leek, and shallot. Sauté for about 10 minutes until the onions, leek, and shallot are a little brown. Add the carrots, celery, thyme, and paprika, and sauté a little longer, stirring to infuse the vegetables with the herbs. Add the tomatoes and the vinegar. Stir to combine. Cover and cook for about 5 minutes. Remove the lid and cook for 3 minutes longer to evaporate the liquid. Add the potatoes, veggie broth, lentils, salt, and pepper to taste. Turn up the heat and bring to a boil. Once boiling, cover the pot with a lid, turn down to a simmer, and cook covered for about 45 minutes or until the lentils are tender.

1 tablespoon extra virgin olive oil or coconut oil

1 large sweet yellow onion, diced

4 cloves garlic, minced

1 leek, white part only, thinly sliced

1 large shallot, diced

3 carrots, peeled and diced

3 stalks celery, chopped small

2 teaspoons dried thyme

1 teaspoon paprika

5 plum tomatoes, diced, or 1 15-ounce can organic fire-roasted diced tomatoes

2 tablespoons champagne vinegar

3 small red potatoes, cut into ¼-inch cubes

6 cups low-sodium vegetable stock or 3 vegetable bouillon cubes and 6 cups water

2 cups French lentils, rinsed and drained

1 teaspoon sea salt

Ground black pepper

**VARIATION**

For added fiber and protein, add 1 cup red lentils to the soup while cooking and increase the water by 1 cup.

# Indian-Spiced Coconut Yam Soup

8 servings

*I love Indian fare and I love yams, so I've combined the two together to make a creamy, delicious soup that will light up your taste buds and transport you right to Marrakesh . . . well, maybe not, but dreaming is fun!*

Heat the oil in a large soup pot over medium heat and sauté the ginger, garlic, celery, and onion until translucent and soft. Add the garam masala and stir to combine to release the flavor of the spice. Add the carrots, yams, and veggie broth. Turn the heat to high and bring to a boil, turn down to a simmer, and cover. Simmer for 20 to 30 minutes or until the yams are soft. Remove from the heat and stir in the coconut milk. Puree using a hand blender until creamy smooth and season with salt and pepper to taste. Top with cinnamon, to taste, before serving.

1 tablespoon coconut oil or extra virgin olive oil

1 teaspoon fresh ground ginger

3 garlic cloves, minced

2 celery stalks, diced

1 medium yellow onion, diced

2 teaspoons garam masala

3 large carrots, diced

3 large garnet yams, peeled and cubed

4 cups vegetable broth or bullion (2 cubes with 4 cups water)

1 15-ounce can coconut milk

Sea salt and cracked black pepper, to taste

Cinnamon

**Karmic Health Tip:** *Coconut oil is loaded with medium-chain fatty acids that help you burn fat and speed up your metabolism, and it is also great to use directly on your skin. I leave a jar in the shower for an après shower smoothing.*

# "Feeling Tropical"
# Black Bean Soup

*This soup transports me right to the turquoise seas
and warm, balmy airs of the Caribbean, one of my favorite
places in the world. I use regular bananas instead of plantains
because they are easier to find. This soup is sweet, spicy,
and oh-so-good. Wear your sunscreen!*

2 tablespoons extra virgin olive oil or coconut oil

1 medium red onion, diced

3 cloves garlic, minced

1 red bell pepper, deseeded and diced

1 green bell pepper, deseeded and diced

1 tablespoon cumin

1 teaspoon ground ginger

¼ teaspoon cayenne pepper

3 15-ounce cans black beans, rinsed and drained

2 ripe bananas, sliced

3 cups vegetable broth

1 15-ounce can coconut milk

Sea salt

Heat the oil in a soup pot over medium heat and sauté the onion, garlic, and red and green bell peppers until soft. Add the cumin, ginger, and cayenne, and stir to combine. Add the black beans, bananas, and vegetable broth. Bring to a boil, then cover, turn down the heat, and simmer about 20 minutes until the fruit is soft. Add the coconut milk and then puree using a blender or stick blender. Add salt to taste. Serve immediately.

 Per Serving: Calories 360, Total Fat 16g, Saturated Fat 11g, Cholesterol 0mg, Sodium 65mg, Carbohydrate 45g, Fiber 14g, Protein 13g

# Kitchen Sink Veggie Soup

*I named this because I make it with any and every vegetable I have in my produce drawer. Hearty, warming, and just what the doctor ordered!*

Heat the oil in a large soup pot over medium heat and sauté the onion, garlic, shallots, and celery until soft. Add the tomatoes and cumin and let the mixture cook down for about 5 minutes. Add the barley (or other grain) and all of the remaining vegetables, along with 4–6 cups of vegetable stock, depending on the size of the soup (you want the liquid to cover the soup by about a ½ inch as it will cook down). Turn up the heat and bring to a boil. Cover and reduce the heat. Simmer until the vegetables are tender, about 20 to 30 minutes, depending on the vegetables used. Season with salt and pepper, to taste, and top with fresh chopped dill or other fresh herbs.

2 tablespoons extra virgin olive oil

1 medium red onion, finely chopped

3 cloves garlic, chopped

2 shallots, chopped

3 celery stalks, chopped small

1 15-ounce can fire-roasted diced tomatoes

2 teaspoons ground cumin

¾ cup barley or any other grain

1 leek, green part removed and white parts thinly sliced

4 carrots, peeled and chopped

4 small red potatoes, diced into ¼-inch cubes

Approximately 6 cups of any combination of seasonal fresh vegetables: zucchini, broccoli, cabbage, cauliflower, yellow squash, green beans (my favorite is garnet yams, Brussels sprouts, cabbage, and zucchini)

4–6 cups vegetable broth (depending on size of soup)

Sea salt and fresh pepper

Any fresh herbs you want (dill, thyme, marjoram, etc.), chopped

## CHEF'S TIP

For a classic veggie soup, use thyme, dill, and marjoram. For Mexican flair, use cilantro and parsley. For an Italian twist, use oregano and thyme.

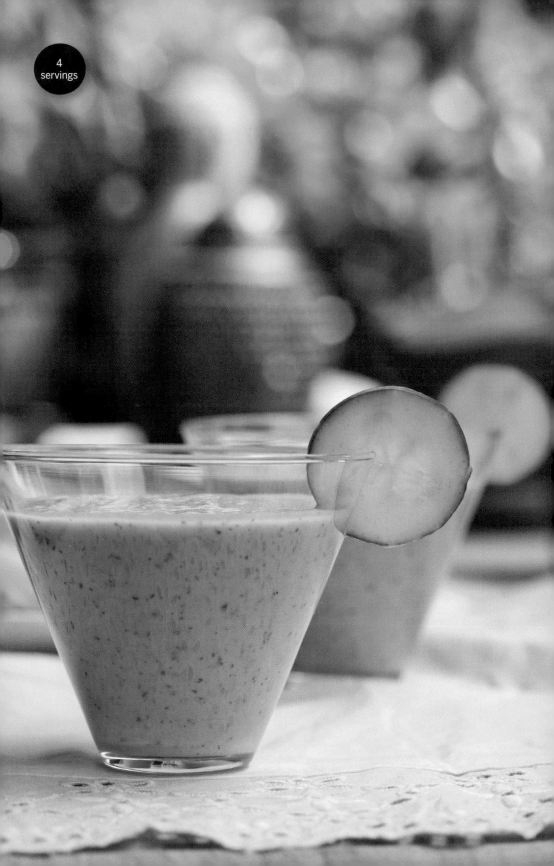

# Holy Moly Green Gazpacho

*This recipe comes from my dear friend and very talented natural food chef, Agi, of One More Bite. She is the connoisseur of gazpacho, and I wouldn't want anyone else's chilled soup in my book but hers! I think you will enjoy this deliciously creamy green concoction on a warm summer day.*

Scoop out the meat of both avocados and place into a blender. Add all of the remaining ingredients except the oil, salt, and pepper. Turn the blender on and let everything mix together. With the motor running, start slowly pouring the oil through the opening in the lid of the blender. This will help emulsify the soup, giving you a light and creamy consistency. Season with salt and pepper. Chill for an hour and enjoy!

2 ripe avocados

2 Persian cucumbers, peeled and diced

1 poblano pepper, deseeded and chopped (if not available, leave out)

1 yellow bell pepper, deseeded and chopped

2 green onions, chopped

¼ cup fresh cilantro

Juice of 2 limes

¼ cup water

⅓ cup extra virgin olive oil

Salt and pepper, to taste

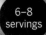
6–8
servings

# Chowdery Corn Soup

*Corn chowder is another classic that is usually made with heavy cream. My plant-based version uses coconut milk, which gives the soup an international flair without so much fat. Eat this with a large salad or veggie wrap for lunch or with some brown rice crisps as an afternoon snack.*

In a soup pot over medium heat, melt the oil and sauté the onion, celery, leek, and garlic until soft. Add the red bell pepper and red pepper flakes. Stir to combine and cook a bit longer, until the bell pepper is soft. Add the yams, potatoes, and broth. Turn the heat to high and bring to a boil. Once boiling, turn down heat, cover, and simmer for about 20 to 30 minutes or until the potatoes are soft. Add the corn and coconut milk and simmer for five more minutes, or until the corn is heated through. Puree the soup with a hand blender, leaving some chunks for texture. Add the chopped cilantro or basil and season with salt and pepper to taste.

1 tablespoon coconut oil

1 medium yellow onion, diced

3 celery stalks, diced

1 leek, white part only, sliced thin

3 garlic cloves, minced

1 red bell pepper, deseeded and diced

¼ teaspoon red pepper flakes

2 large garnet yams, peeled and cubed

3 red bliss baby potatoes, cubed

4 cups vegetable broth (or 2 bouillon cubes with 4 cups water)

110-ounce bag organic sweet white frozen corn

1 15-ounce can coconut milk (full fat is preferred, but you can use lite)

Handful of freshly chopped cilantro or basil

Sea salt and pepper, to taste

# Golden Split Pea Soup

*Split pea soup is an all-time classic, and this is my veganized version using sunny yellow split peas! If you can't find liquid smoke in your grocery store, just leave it out, although it does give the soup the smoky ham flavor that most split pea soups contain.*

1 tablespoon extra virgin olive oil

1 medium yellow onion, diced

3 stalks celery, diced

1 leek, halved and cut in thin slices, white parts only

4 carrots, diced

4 red potatoes, cut in ½-inch cubes

2 teaspoons chopped fresh thyme or 1 teaspoon dried thyme

2 teaspoons chopped fresh marjoram or 1 teaspoon dried marjoram

2 cups yellow split peas

6 cups vegetable broth

1 teaspoon sea salt or to taste

Freshly ground pepper

⅛ teaspoon liquid smoke (optional)

Heat the oil in a large stockpot over medium heat and sauté the onion, celery, and leek until soft and translucent. Add the carrots, potatoes, thyme, and marjoram, and stir well. Add the split peas and broth and stir to combine. Bring to a boil, then cover and lower heat to a simmer. Cook for about 30 to 45 minutes or until split peas are soft and mushy. Add the salt, pepper, and liquid smoke, if using, to taste. You can serve as is or puree this soup using a hand blender if you like a creamier soup.

## CHEF'S TIP

If you are not able to find golden split peas in your grocery store, green ones will do just fine.

Per Serving: Calories 410, Total Fat 3g, Saturated Fat 0g, Cholesterol 0mg, Sodium 610mg, Carbohydrate 78g, Fiber 6g, Protein 21g

# Cream of Celery Soup

*Celery is not often the star of its very own dish, so I created this soup to feature this hydrating, calming veggie that is loaded with potassium and minerals. I think you will love this soup, and you won't even miss the cream, I promise. It's awesome to make around holiday time to calm your nerves—or anytime, really!*

Heat the oil in a large soup pot over medium heat and sauté the onion, garlic, and leek until soft. Add the celery seed, thyme, and sea salt, and stir well to release the flavor of the herbs. Cook for about 2 to 3 minutes, stirring occasionally. Add the carrots and celery and cook for 5 minutes longer until the celery starts to soften. Add the potatoes, vegetable broth, and bay leaves. Turn up the heat to high, cover, and bring to a boil. Once boiling, turn down to a simmer and cook for about 20 to 30 minutes until the potatoes are soft. Puree the soup using a hand blender or a regular blender until creamy smooth. Add the coconut milk. Stir well and season with pepper.

2 tablespoons olive oil

1 large sweet yellow onion, diced

1 tablespoon minced garlic

1 leek, white parts only, thinly sliced

½ teaspoon celery seed

1 teaspoon thyme

1¼ teaspoons sea salt

3 carrots, peeled and coarsely chopped

8 stalks celery, chopped (including the leaves)

4 small red potatoes, scrubbed, then chopped with skins on

5 cups vegetable broth

2 bay leaves

1 cup coconut milk or plain almond milk

Freshly cracked pepper, to taste

# Dreamy Roasted Butternut Squash Soup

*I love the fall because squash is in season, and butternut is one of my faves! This soup is so good you will want to eat the whole pot —that's why I termed it "dreamy." Top with some lightly toasted pumpkin seeds right before serving for presentation, crunch, and a little extra calcium and magnesium.*

1 large butternut squash, roasted (this can be done a day before serving)

2 tablespoons olive oil or coconut oil

1 large shallot, diced small

½ large yellow sweet onion, diced

1-inch piece fresh ginger, peeled and grated

1 large garnet yam or sweet potato, peeled and cubed

2 stalks celery, diced

5 carrots, peeled and chopped

½ teaspoon cumin powder

4 cups vegetable broth

2 tablespoons agave nectar or maple syrup

Sea salt and pepper, to taste

1 teaspoon cinnamon

¼ teaspoon nutmeg

Pinch of cloves

1½ cups unsweetened almond milk or coconut milk

Toasted pumpkin seeds (for garnish)

Heat the oven to 400 degrees F. Cut squash in half lengthwise. Line a baking dish or cookie sheet with parchment paper and lightly coat with cooking spray (olive oil or coconut). Place the squash cut side down on the baking dish or sheet and poke holes in it with a sharp knife or fork, then spray squash with cooking spray. Bake for about 45 minutes or until the squash can be easily pierced with a fork. Take out of the oven and let it cool.

Heat the oil in a large pot over medium heat. Add the shallot, onion, and ginger,

Per Serving: Calories 170, Total Fat 4.5g, Saturated Fat 0.5g, Cholesterol 0mg, Sodium 260mg, Carbohydrate 32g, Fiber 5g, Protein 3g

and sauté for about 3 minutes until soft and translucent. Add the yam, celery, and carrots. Sauté for a few minutes and then add the cumin powder, stirring to incorporate. Add the broth. Cover the pot and bring to a boil. Turn down the heat and simmer until the vegetables are tender, about 20 minutes.

While the soup is cooking, remove the seeds from the squash and discard. Scoop out the flesh from the skin and add to the pot, stirring to incorporate the squash with the other vegetables. Add a bit more broth if necessary. Cook for about 5 more minutes, then remove from the heat and add the agave nectar, salt and pepper, cinnamon, nutmeg, cloves, and the almond milk. Puree the soup using a hand blender or in batches in a regular blender. Serve garnished with toasted pumpkin seeds.

*Did You Know?* Maple syrup is chock-full of vitamins and minerals. Make sure to buy grade B, which is the most nutritious and least processed. It's a low-glycemic sweetener, so it won't spike your blood sugar as fast as some other sweeteners.

# Curried Veggie "Stoup"

*"Stoup" is a stew and a soup all in one. Enjoy this flavorful curry dish in a large bowl scooped over a bed of quinoa or basmati rice. It's a hearty meal in itself. Delish!*

3 tablespoons coconut oil

1 shallot, diced

2 garlic cloves, finely diced

½ large yellow onion, chopped

2 teaspoons fresh grated ginger

4 tablespoons curry powder

1 head of cauliflower, chopped into bite-size pieces

1 cup broccoli florets

1 large green apple, peeled and chopped

3 carrots, peeled and chopped

1 parsnip, peeled and chopped

1 large garnet yam, peeled and cut into ½-inch cubes

1.06 quarts (1 liter) vegetable stock (or 2 vegetable bouillon cubes dissolved in 4 cups boiling water)

2 cups fresh baby spinach

1 15-ounce can coconut milk

1 tablespoon grade B maple syrup or raw agave nectar

Juice of one lime

1 handful fresh basil, chopped (optional)

Salt and pepper, to taste

In a large stockpot, heat the coconut oil over medium heat and sauté the shallot, garlic, onion, and ginger until translucent, about 5 minutes. Add the curry powder and stir well to incorporate, sautéing for about 2 minutes more. Add the cauliflower and broccoli, and stir to coat with the seasoning. Add the apple, carrots, parsnip, and yam, and stir together. Pour in the vegetable stock, raise the heat, and bring to a boil. Put the lid on, lower the heat, and simmer for 20 minutes or until the vegetables are cooked through. Remove from the heat and then add the spinach and allow it to wilt down, about 2 minutes. Add the coconut milk, maple syrup, lime juice, basil, and salt and pepper to taste. Let the stoup sit for 5 minutes before serving.

# Kinda Like Mom's Beefy Stew

*Well, not really, but it's my special version of "beef" stew, and I find it to be tasty, simple to make, and a favorite with kids as well!*

Heat the olive oil in a stockpot over medium heat. Add the onion and celery and sauté until the onion is translucent. Add the tempeh, oregano, and Worcestershire sauce and cook for a few more minutes until the tempeh is infused with flavors. Add the yams, carrots, and parsnips, and stir to combine. Cook for 3 minutes and then add the vegetable broth, tomatoes (break them up with your hand or a spoon), bay leaf, and brown rice. Stir together to combine well. Bring to a boil and then cover the pot and simmer until all of the vegetables and the rice are tender, about 20 minutes. Add the frozen peas and stir to combine. Remove from the heat and let it sit for 5 minutes so the peas "cook." Serve immediately!

- 2 tablespoons extra virgin olive oil
- 2 cups diced red onions (about 2 medium onions)
- 1 cup chopped celery (with leaves)
- 2 8-ounce packages tempeh, cut into ¼-inch cubes
- 1 teaspoon dried oregano
- 1 tablespoon vegan Worcestershire sauce
- 4 cups peeled and cubed garnet yams (about 2 medium yams)
- 4 large carrots, cut into ¼-inch sliced rounds
- 3 medium parsnips, peeled and cubed
- 4 cups vegetable broth
- 1 28-ounce can fire-roasted whole tomatoes in juice
- 1 bay leaf
- ¾ cup short-grain brown rice or barley, rinsed
- 1½ cups frozen peas

**Did You Know?** Soup for breakfast? Yes—you betcha! I love having soup for breakfast. Think about it: It's nutritious, warming, and light. It's a great way to start off the day. Think outside the breakfast box!

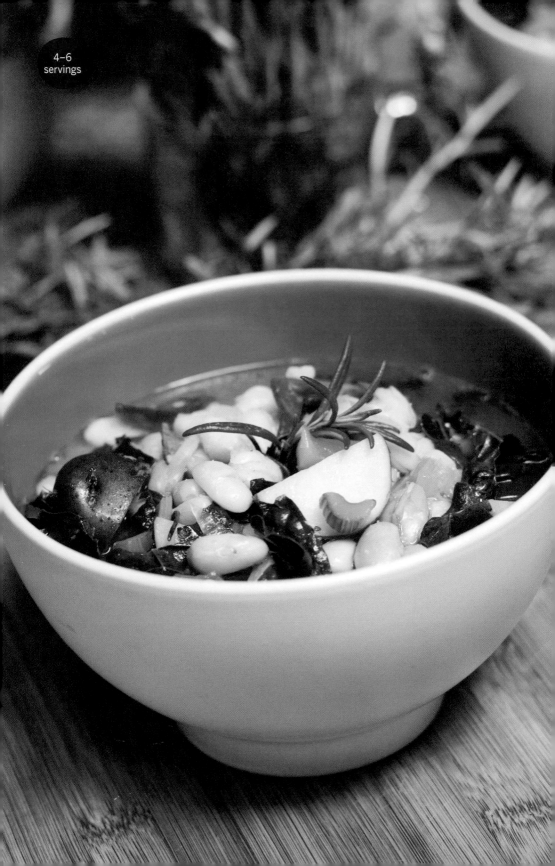

4–6
servings

# Garlicky White Bean and Kale Soup

*Garlic and kale are two of my favorite foods . . . seriously.*
*Garlic is great for the immune system and the heart, and kale is*
*one of the most nutrient-dense foods you can eat. These two combined*
*create a powwow of immune-boosting flavors that will*
*dance on your tongue and warm your belly.*

Heat the olive oil in a large soup pot over medium heat and sauté the garlic, onion, and celery until soft. Add the tomatoes, sherry vinegar, and rosemary and let it cook for a few minutes until the vinegar evaporates. Add the bay leaf, beans, kale, potatoes, and veggie broth and bring to a boil. Turn down to a simmer, cover, and cook for about 25 minutes or until the potatoes are soft. Remove from the heat and dissolve the miso paste into the soup by stirring in. Add the nutritional yeast and season with salt and pepper, if needed. Serve immediately.

2 tablespoons extra virgin olive oil

8 cloves of garlic, minced

1 large sweet yellow onion, diced

2 stalks celery, diced

4 roma tomatoes, roughly chopped

1 tablespoon sherry vinegar

2 teaspoons freshly chopped rosemary

1 bay leaf

3 15-ounce cans white beans, drained and rinsed

½ bunch kale, chopped into small pieces (Lacinato kale is best in this soup)

4 small red potatoes, diced into ½-inch cubes

5 cups veggie broth

1 tablespoon mellow white miso

1 tablespoon nutritional yeast

Sea salt and freshly ground pepper, to taste

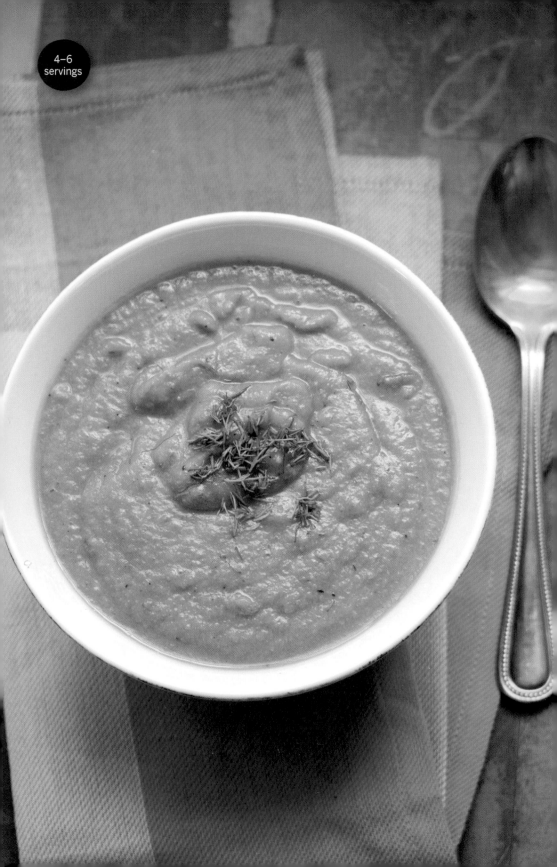

# Dill-icious Roasted Carrot Cauliflower Soup

*This soup is so fresh-tasting, and I love the golden orange color of it once it is pureed. It's light, nutritious, and great to pair with a salad for lunch!*

Preheat the oven to 400 degrees F. Place the cauliflower and carrots in a large bowl and drizzle with olive oil. Toss to coat and spread out on a cookie sheet lined with parchment paper. Roast until soft, about 20 minutes. In the meantime, heat the oil in a large soup pot over medium heat. Sauté the onion and garlic until soft. Add the roasted cauliflower, carrots, and the veggie broth. Simmer over medium heat for about 10 minutes. Puree using a hand blender or regular blender. Add the maple syrup and fresh dill and season with salt and pepper. Stir well and serve immediately.

- 1 medium head cauliflower, chopped into bite-size pieces
- 2 pounds carrots, peeled and chopped into ½-inch pieces
- 2 tablespoons extra virgin olive oil (plus extra for drizzling) or coconut oil
- 1 large yellow onion, diced
- 4 cloves garlic, peeled and coarsely chopped
- 5 cups vegetable broth
- 2 teaspoons maple syrup
- 2 tablespoons finely chopped fresh dill
- Sea salt and pepper, to taste

**CHEF'S TIP**

If you don't have time to buy fresh dill or you can't find it, you can substitute dried dill, but use half the amount. Your soup will still be good, but won't taste as dill-icious as it would with fresh.

# Smoky Tempeh Chili

*This veganized version of chili is much healthier for you and it still has tons of flavor! It's great to take to a potluck or Super Bowl party. Just for fun, don't even tell your guests it's meat free, and see what they say after a mouthful. I guarantee they won't even miss the meat.*

2 tablespoons olive oil

1 medium red onion, diced

3 cloves garlic, diced

2 red bell peppers, deseeded and diced

1 8-ounce package tempeh, crumbled

2 tablespoons chili powder blend or chipotle chili powder (if you like it spicy)

1 teaspoon ground coriander

1 teaspoon ground cumin

1 teaspoon dried oregano

2 15-ounce cans fire-roasted diced tomatoes

1 cup water

1 15-ounce can black beans, drained and rinsed

1 15-ounce can red kidney beans, drained and rinsed

1 15-ounce can white beans, drained and rinsed

1 cup frozen corn

Cooked brown rice (optional)

Freshly chopped cilantro for garnish (optional)

Heat the olive oil in a stockpot over medium heat and sauté the red onion, garlic, and red bell peppers. Once soft, crumble in the tempeh and add the chili powder, coriander, cumin, and oregano. Cook for a few minutes, stirring to incorporate the tempeh with all the spices. Add the tomatoes, water, and beans. Cover and simmer for about 30 minutes. Add the corn and cook a few more minutes until the corn is soft. Serve over brown rice and top with cilantro, if desired.

Per Serving: Calories 430, Total Fat 10g, Saturated Fat 2g, Cholesterol 0mg, Sodium 440mg, Carbohydrate 62g, Fiber 17g, Protein 25g

# Chapter 4

# *Succulent Salads and Delicious Dressings*

**S**alads are honestly one of my favorite dishes. I love to turn them into a meal by adding beans, nuts, tons of veggies, and grains. I also enjoy eating them alongside other dishes to complete a meal. Eating a raw salad every day will ensure that you are getting lots of nutrients and healthy enzymes in your body; they are also high in fiber and will fill you up, which can help prevent overeating. Making your own salad dressing is a snap, so there is no reason to buy bottled salad dressing that is usually high in sugar and fat. Make the dressings in batches and keep in the refrigerator to grab any time you whip up a salad.

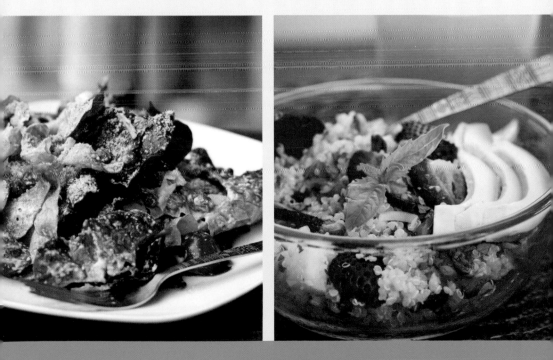

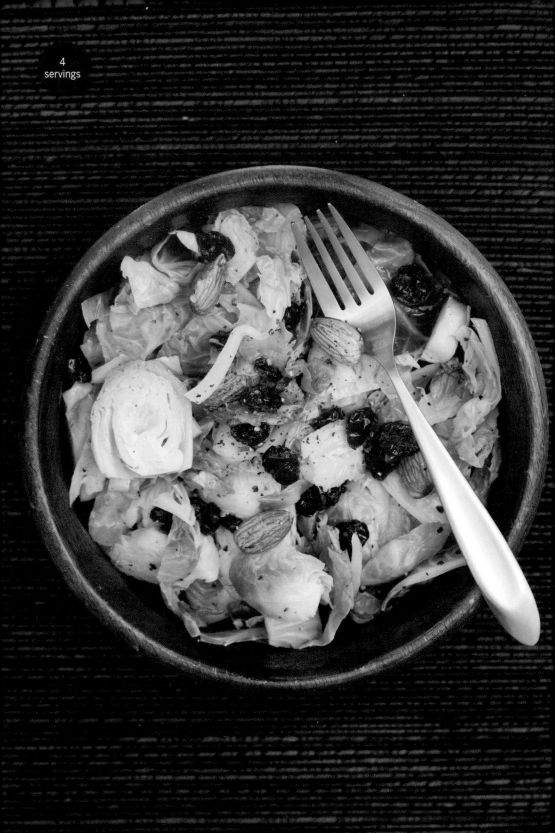

# Brussels Sprouts Salad

*If you are not a fan of Brussels sprouts yet, I promise you will be after eating this delicious and surprising salad. Brussels sprouts are a great cancer-fighting food because they are loaded with antioxidants and they help to detoxify the body.*

Blanch the Brussels sprouts in boiling water for 3 minutes. Drain and set aside to cool. Once cool, place in a bowl and add the almonds, cranberries, and shallots. Toss with vinaigrette (recipe follows). Season with salt and pepper. This salad gets more flavorful if refrigerated overnight to allow the flavors to meld together.

1 pound Brussels sprouts, ends cut off and then thinly sliced

½ cup almonds (smoked or roasted)

½ cup dried cranberries

1 large shallot, diced

Lemon Vinaigrette (see recipe below)

Sea salt and pepper, to taste

## Lemon Vinaigrette

Juice of 1 lemon

2 tablespoons extra virgin olive oil

3 tablespoons brown rice vinegar

1 teaspoon agave nectar

1 tablespoon Dijon mustard (I prefer Annie's Organics or Trader Joe's brands)

1 shallot, minced finely

This snazzy vinaigrette is great on any type of salad. Make some extra and store it in your fridge to have on hand whenever you need a dressing.

Place all of the ingredients in a blender or shaker bottle and blend or shake until well mixed.

Per Serving: Calories 210, Total Fat 10g, Saturated Fat 1g, Cholesterol 0mg, Sodium 30mg, Carbohydrate 28g, Fiber 7g, Protein 8g
Lemon Vinaigrette: Calories 80, Total Fat 7g, Saturated Fat 1g, Cholesterol 0mg, Sodium 90mg, Carbohydrate 5g, Fiber 0g, Protein 0g

115

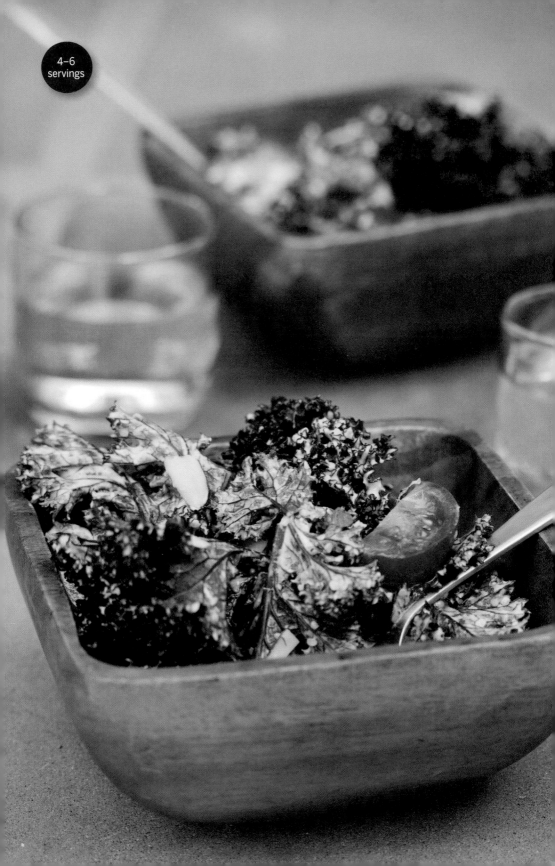

# Raw Kale Salad
# with Creamy Chipotle Dressing

*This salad is a hit with many of my clients.
It turned them into kale converts, and now they request it
every time I cook for them! I think you will love the smokiness of
the dressing combined with the curly leaves of the kale.*

Strip the kale of stems, tear into small pieces, and soak in a bowl with water for a few minutes to get rid of any sand or dirt. Drain the kale and dry using a salad spinner. Place the kale in a large bowl and drizzle with the olive oil and a dash of salt. Massage the kale with your hands for a few minutes until it softens, which helps the kale become easier to digest. Add the tomatoes, almonds, and hemp seeds and toss with the Chipotle Dressing (recipe follows).

1 or 2 heads kale, any variety (I like curly kale for this salad)

Extra virgin olive oil, roughly 2 teaspoons

Dash of sea salt

½ cup quartered or halved cherry tomatoes

¼ cup slivered almonds

3 tablespoons hemp seeds

## Creamy Chipotle Dressing
**(About ½ cup)**

¼ cup tahini

2 tablespoons extra virgin olive oil

3 tablespoons apple cider vinegar

2 tablespoons agave nectar

2 tablespoons filtered water

Juice of 1 lemon

⅛ teaspoon chipotle chili powder

Blend all of the ingredients together in a blender or Magic Bullet until smooth and creamy. This dressing will be thick. If you like a thinner dressing, add 1 to 2 tablespoons of water and reblend.

Per Serving: Calories 110, Total Fat 6g, Saturated Fat 0.5g, Cholesterol 0mg, Sodium 35mg, Carbohydrate 10g, Fiber 2g, Protein 5g
Creamy Chipotle Dressing: Calories 120, Total Fat 10g, Saturated Fat 1.5g, Cholesterol 0mg, Sodium 0mg,
Carbohydrate 8g, Fiber 0g, Protein 2g

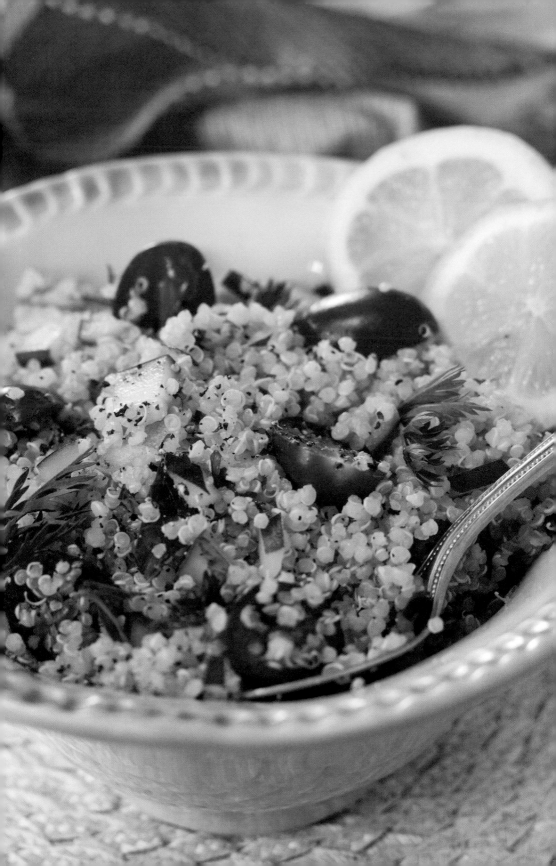

# Quinoa Tabbouleh

6 servings

*A different twist on the classic Mediterranean dish using quinoa instead of bulgur wheat, which results in a gluten-free dish! I love to serve this with a dollop of hummus and some olives on the side to make it even more heart healthy.*

Cook quinoa according to the package directions. Once cooked, transfer to a large bowl to cool. Combine the quinoa with the remaining ingredients and stir to combine. Season with salt and pepper.

1 cup quinoa

¼ cup chopped fresh mint

½ cup chopped fresh parsley

1 cup peeled and diced cucumber

1 cup halved cherry tomatoes

2 tablespoons extra virgin olive oil

2 garlic cloves, minced

¼ cup lemon juice

Sea salt and black pepper, to taste

**Did You Know?** Wild rice is really not rice at all but a species of grass that grows in slow-flowing streams and the shallow water in lakes. Some Native American tribes, such as the Ojibwe, consider wild rice a sacred part of their culture. It is high in fiber, protein, and lysine, contains minerals and B vitamins, and is naturally gluten free.

# Wild Rice Salad with Balsamic Maple Dressing

*Wild rice and spelt berries combine to give this salad a pleasing and chewy texture. When you add dried cherries, scallions, pecans, and grapes, you have a delicious amalgamation of flavors that your taste buds will love!*

Cook the wild rice and spelt berries as per package directions. Once cooked, place both into a large bowl. Stir in the sea salt, onion, scallions, pecans, dried cherries, and grapes. Add the Balsamic Maple Dressing (recipe follows).

To make this dish gluten-free, replace the spelt berries with regular short-grain brown rice.

1 cup wild rice blend, rinsed

½ cup spelt berries

½ teaspoon sea salt

½ cup finely diced red onion

4 scallions, green parts removed, thinly sliced

¼ cup chopped pecans

½ cup dried cherries

1 cup red grapes, halved

## Balsamic Maple Dressing

1 garlic clove, crushed

½ teaspoon sea salt

3 tablespoons balsamic vinegar

1 tablespoon stone-ground mustard

1 tablespoon maple syrup

⅓ cup extra virgin olive oil

¼ teaspoon fresh ground pepper

Place all of the ingredients together in a small bowl and whisk to combine. Stir the dressing into the grains and let the salad sit for a few minutes to marry the flavors. Serve warm or at room temperature. (Making the dressing the day before allows more time for the flavors to blend. If you like, you can warm it up before serving.)

Per Serving: Calories 370, Total Fat 7g, Saturated Fat 0g, Cholesterol 0mg, Sodium 10mg, Carbohydrate 75g, Fiber 8g, Protein 8g
Balsamic Maple Dressing: Calories 190, Total Fat 18g, Saturated Fat 2.5g, Cholesterol 0mg, Sodium 350mg, Carbohydrate 6g, Fiber 0g, Protein 0g

# Dilled Potato Salad

*Who doesn't love potato salad (especially when it's made with lower-sugar bliss potatoes and heart-healthy grapeseed Vegenaise)? If you can't find Vegenaise at your grocery store, any vegan mayo will do. When using the red, purple, and yellow variety of potatoes, you will have a festive red, white, and blue combo worthy of any Fourth of July picnic table. It's sure to be a hit with your friends.*

3 pounds red bliss potatoes or a combination of red, purple, and creamy yellow potatoes, unpeeled and chopped into ½-inch bites

1 small red onion, finely diced

4 scallions, white parts only, thinly sliced

3 tablespoons freshly chopped dill

¼ cup grapeseed Vegenaise

1 tablespoon Dijon mustard (I prefer Whole Foods, Annie's, or Trader Joe's brands)

2 teaspoons freshly squeezed lemon juice

1 tablespoon apple cider vinegar

Sea salt and pepper, to taste

Boil the potatoes until tender but not too soft, about 15 to 20 minutes. Drain and cool. In a large bowl, combine the potatoes with the remaining ingredients and stir to combine. Season with salt and pepper. Cover and refrigerate until cold, at least 3 hours. If the salad becomes dry after a day or two, add a bit more Vegenaise.

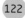 Per Serving: Calories 170, Total Fat 5g, Saturated Fat 1g, Cholesterol 0mg, Sodium 120mg, Carbohydrate 29g, Fiber 3g, Protein 3g

# Herb-Infused Chickpea Salad

4 servings

*Chickpeas are loaded with protein and fiber.*
*I combined them here with some delicious baby artichokes*
*and fresh herbs for a delightful blend of flavors.*
*This salad is best served when it's warm.*

Place chickpeas and sundried tomatoes in a large bowl. Set aside. Heat the olive oil in a skillet over medium heat. Sauté the onion, garlic, and celery until tender and slightly caramelized. Add the artichoke hearts and sauté until lightly browned. Add the mixture to the chickpeas and sundried tomatoes and stir well to combine. Top with Herbed Lemon Dressing (recipe follows).

2 15-ounce cans chickpeas or
   3 cups cooked chickpeas

¼ cup sliced sundried tomatoes

2 tablespoons extra virgin olive oil

1 small red onion, diced

4 garlic cloves, diced

1 celery stalk, diced

12 artichokes hearts, cut into
   quarters

### Herbed Lemon Dressing

3 tablespoons fresh lemon juice

¼ cup extra virgin olive oil

1 tablespoon finely chopped fresh
   dill or rosemary

Salt and pepper, to taste

Put all of the dressing ingredients into a small bowl and whisk until combined. Pour over the chickpea salad and stir to combine flavors. Let the salad sit for a few minutes and serve slightly warm.

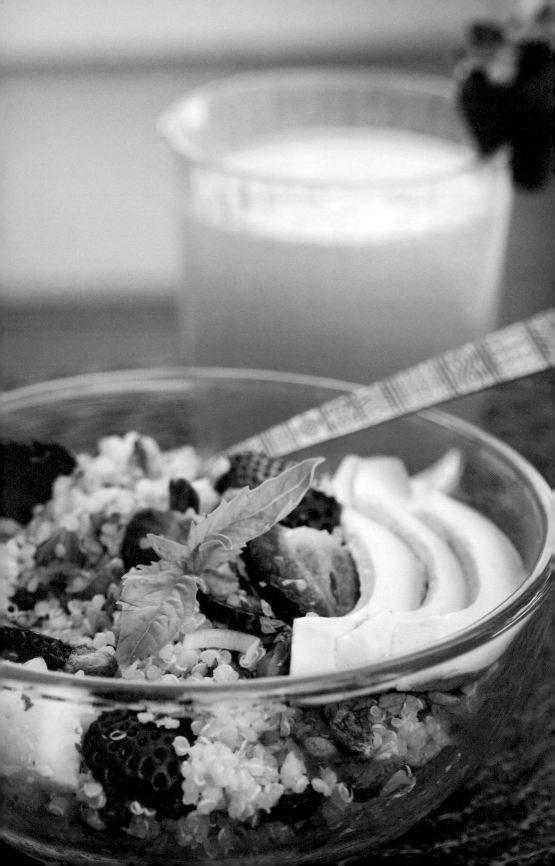

# Quinoa and Strawberry Salad with Lime Vinaigrette

6–8 servings

*This salad is high in protein, loaded with flavor and texture, and perfect to serve for lunch on a warm summer afternoon.*

Cook the quinoa according to package directions and set aside to cool. Combine remaining ingredients in a large bowl and drizzle with the Lime Vinaigrette (recipe follows). Stir to combine.

1 cup quinoa, rinsed, cooked, and cooled

1 cup hulled and quartered strawberries

½ cup peeled and diced jicama

1 avocado, peeled and diced

2 scallions, thinly sliced

2 tablespoons freshly chopped mint

3 tablespoons dry-roasted pistachios

## Lime Vinaigrette

¼ cup extra virgin olive oil

3 tablespoons lime juice

2 tablespoons brown rice vinegar

2 teaspoons Dijon mustard

2 teaspoons agave nectar

Pinch of sea salt

Mix all of the dressing ingredients in a blender or shaker bottle until well combined.

Per Serving: Calories 140, Total Fat 5g, Saturated Fat 0.5g, Cholesterol 0mg, Sodium 15mg, Carbohydrate 19g, Fiber 3g, Protein 5g

Lime Vinaigrette: Per Serving: Calories 70, Total Fat 7g, Saturated Fat 1g, Cholesterol 0mg, Sodium 30mg, Carbohydrate 3g, Fiber 0g, Protein 0g

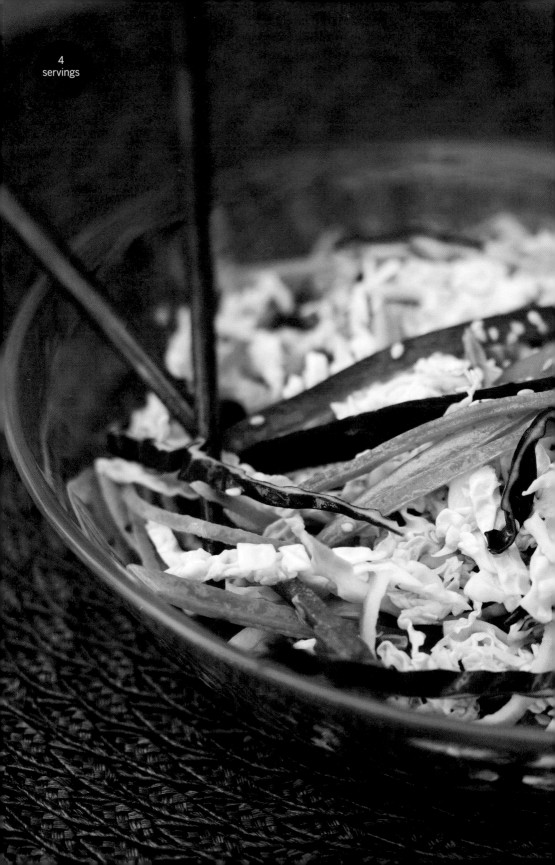

# Raw Thai Slaw

*I love this Asian version of coleslaw because it's light,
fresh, and great to serve alongside a sandwich or as a side
to any meal. If you cannot find Napa cabbage,
use white cabbage instead.*

Combine all of the ingredients for the slaw in a large bowl. Blend the dressing ingredients together in a blender or shaker bottle and pour over the slaw. Toss well to combine. Refrigerate at least 2 hours so the flavors meld.

1 medium head Napa cabbage, shredded

½ small head red cabbage, shredded

½ small red onion, thinly sliced

1 red bell pepper, deseeded and julienned

½ cup julienned snow peas

½ cup shredded carrots

2 tablespoons chopped peanuts

## Thai Dressing

3 tablespoons toasted sesame oil

3 tablespoons rice wine vinegar

1 tablespoon ume plum vinegar (optional)

1 tablespoon agave nectar or maple syrup

Juice from ½ lime

Pinch red pepper flakes

Per Serving: Calories 70, Total Fat 2.5g, Saturated Fat 0g, Cholesterol 0mg, Sodium 25mg, Carbohydrate 10g, Fiber 3g, Protein 3g
Thai Dressing: Calories 110, Total Fat 10g, Saturated Fat 1.5g, Cholesterol 0mg, Sodium 0mg, Carbohydrate 5g, Fiber 0g, Protein 0g

127

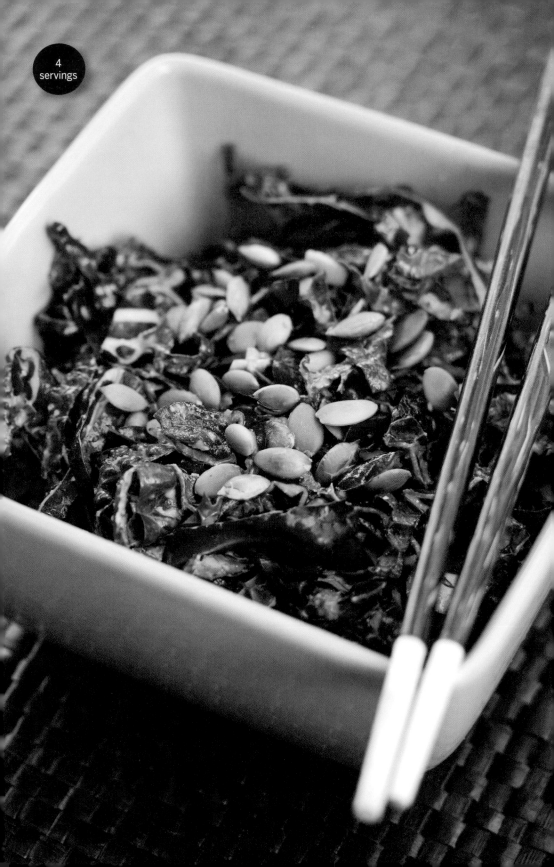

# Kale Slaw with Creamy Pumpkin Seed Dressing

*This is another favorite recipe from natural food chef, Agi G, of One More Bite. I fell in love with this slaw at one of her dinner parties, and I begged her for the recipe to add to my book. I'm sure you will really love it, too . . . it's crunchy, creamy, and slightly sweet.*

Place the chopped kale, cabbage, and cranberries in a large bowl. Put the dressing ingredients into a blender (or Magic Bullet) and blend until combined into a smooth and creamy consistency. Pour the dressing over the salad and toss. Cover with plastic wrap and let it chill in the refrigerator for at least 30 minutes. Right before serving, sprinkle the salad with the remaining toasted pepitas.

2 cups chopped fresh organic kale (stems removed)

2 cups shredded white (or red) cabbage

¼ cup dried cranberries

1 tablespoon toasted pepitas (Spanish pumpkin seeds) for garnish

## Creamy Pumpkin Seed Dressing

3 tablespoons toasted pepitas (Spanish pumpkin seeds)

2 tablespoons of water

2–3 tablespoons lemon juice

⅓ cup extra virgin olive oil

1 tablespoon raw honey or maple syrup

1 tablespoon of Dijon mustard

Pinch of sea salt

Pinch of black pepper

Per Serving: Calories 60, Total Fat 1.5g, Saturated Fat 0g, Cholesterol 0mg, Sodium 20mg, Carbohydrate 12g, Fiber 2g, Protein 2g
Creamy Pumpkin Seed Dressing: Per Serving: Calories 220, Total Fat 21g, Saturated Fat 3g, Cholesterol 0mg, Sodium 90mg, Carbohydrate 5g, Fiber 0g, Protein 2g

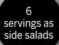

## CHEF'S TIP

Tempeh bacon can be found in the refrigerated specialty items section near the tofu and nondairy milk. If you cannot find tempeh bacon, just leave it out; this salad is just as good without it.

# Spinach Salad with "Bacon" and Creamy Tahini Dressing

*This version of spinach salad reminds me of the one I used to eat back in my meat-eating days with crunchy, smoky bacon and creamy dressing. Hemp seeds add an extra punch of fiber and are high in omega-3s (larger amount than walnuts), omega-6s, omega-9s, vitamins (especially B), and protein.*

Place all of the ingredients for the salad in a large bowl. Blend all of the ingredients for the dressing in a blender or Magic Bullet until smooth and pour over salad mixture.

6 cups baby spinach leaves, stems removed (if the stems are extra-long or dirty)

¼ cup pine nuts

4 pieces tempeh bacon, browned and broken into small pieces (Light Life brand is my favorite)

½ cup halved cherry tomatoes

3 tablespoons hemp seeds

¼ cup thinly sliced red onion

1 cup chickpeas, rinsed and drained

## Creamy Tahini Dressing

¼ cup tahini

1 tablespoon water

2 tablespoons apple cider vinegar

2 teaspoons tamari or Braggs Aminos

1 tablespoon lemon juice

2 tablespoons extra virgin olive oil, flaxseed oil, or untoasted sesame oil

1 tablespoon sweet mellow white miso

1 date, pitted, or 1 tablespoon maple syrup

1 clove garlic, finely minced

Per Serving: Calories 140, Total Fat 7g, Saturated Fat 0.5g, Cholesterol 0mg, Sodium 135mg, Carbohydrate 13g, Fiber 4g, Protein 7g
Creamy Tahini Dressing: Per Serving: Calories 120, Total Fat 10g, Saturated Fat 1.5g, Cholesterol 0mg, Sodium 130mg, Carbohydrate 6g, Fiber 1g, Protein 2g

# White Bean Zucchini Salad

*This is a great summer salad when zucchini is growing like weeds.*
*It's light, flavorful, and great as a side salad*
*to complement any meal.*

½ medium yellow onion, diced

2 shallots, diced

1 tablespoon extra virgin olive oil

1 teaspoon dried thyme

½ teaspoon dried sage

½ teaspoon dried marjoram

2 large zucchini, cut in half lengthwise and sliced into ¼-inch pieces

1 cup chopped baby spinach

¼ cup sundried tomatoes, marinated in oil, drained, and thinly sliced

2 15-ounce cans white beans, drained and rinsed

Sea salt and pepper, to taste

In a large skillet over medium heat, sauté the onion and shallot in olive oil until translucent and caramelized. Add the thyme, sage, and marjoram, and stir to combine and release the flavor of the herbs. Add the zucchini and sauté until lightly browned. Pour into a large bowl with the spinach, tomatoes, and beans, and stir well to combine. Season with salt and pepper. Serve warm or chilled.

Per Serving: Calories 110, Total Fat 2.5g, Saturated Fat 0g, Cholesterol 0mg, Sodium 20mg, Carbohydrate 18g, Fiber 4g, Protein 6g

# Mixed Baby Greens with Walnut, Pear, and Pomegranate Mint Dressing

*Baby greens salads are my favorite and also the most versatile. This version looks very elegant to serve at a luncheon or dinner party. It's a delightful version that is fresh, minty, and loaded with nutrition, texture, and sweetness.*

Place all of the ingredients for the salad into a large bowl. Blend the dressing ingredients in a blender or Magic Bullet until smooth. Pour over the salad ingredients and toss until salad is well mixed. Serve immediately.

6 cups baby greens mix

1 Bosc pear, cored and thinly sliced

¼ cup dried cranberries (fruit-juice sweetened are best)

⅓ cup chopped toasted walnuts or hazelnuts

½ cup thinly sliced red onion

¼ cup pomegranate seeds (optional)

### Pomegranate Mint Dressing

3 tablespoons pomegranate juice, preferably fresh squeezed or not from concentrate

2 tablespoons flaxseed oil or extra virgin olive oil

1 tablespoon agave nectar

2 tablespoons apple cider vinegar

1 tablespoon Dijon mustard

Sea salt, to taste

Per Serving: Calories 140, Total Fat 4g, Saturated Fat 0g, Cholesterol 0mg, Sodium 600mg, Carbohydrate 18g, Fiber 6g, Protein 6g
Pomegranate Mint Dressing: Per Serving: Calories 60, Total Fat 4.5g, Saturated Fat 0.5g, Cholesterol 0mg, Sodium 60mg, Carbohydrate 4g, Fiber 0g, Protein 0g

# Vegan Caesar Salad

**3–4 servings**

*Caesar salad is one of my favorite salads, but the normal version is usually high in fat. I think you will really enjoy this light, tasty version, and you won't even miss the Parmesan cheese. Top with some gluten-free croutons for extra crunch.*

## Salad

1 large head romaine lettuce, cleaned and chopped

½ cup halved cherry tomatoes

3 tablespoons capers

¼ cup thinly sliced red onion

2 tablespoons Vegan Parmesan

## Caesar Dressing

2 tablespoons apple cider vinegar

½ cup raw cashews

3 tablespoons nutritional yeast

1 tablespoon hemp seeds

10 walnuts

¼ cup fresh lemon juice

2 dates, pitted

¼ cup extra virgin olive oil

2 cloves garlic

1 teaspoon sea salt

Fresh ground black pepper to taste

¼ cup water

Place salad ingredients, except for Vegan Parmesan, in a large bowl. Combine the dressing ingredients in a blender and process until smooth and creamy. Drizzle the dressing over the top of the salad and toss with tongs until the mixture is well combined. Dressing will be thick, so you can add more water to it if you prefer a thinner dressing. Put the Parmesan ingredients in a blender or small food processor and blend until combined (it will be a bit chunky). Top the salad with the Vegan Parmesan and serve.

## Vegan Parmesan

½ cup toasted walnuts

3 tablespoons nutritional yeast

¼ teaspoon sea salt

Per Serving: Calories 80, Total Fat 3.5g, Saturated Fat 0g, Cholesterol 0mg, Sodium 260mg, Carbohydrate 9g, Fiber 5g, Protein 5g
Caesar Dressing: Calories 260, Total Fat 22g, Saturated Fat 3g, Cholesterol 0mg, Sodium 590mg, Carbohydrate 12g, Fiber 3g, Protein 6g
Vegan Parmesan: Per Serving: Calories 150, Total Fat 12g, Saturated Fat 0.5g, Cholesterol 0mg, Sodium 190mg, Carbohydrate 4g, Fiber 3g, Protein 9g

# Chapter 5

# Main Dish Favorites: Veganized

*T*his chapter contains all of my favorite main dishes, veganized. Burgers, pasta, meatballs, burritos—you name it, it's here. All of these dishes are loaded with flavor and texture and are simple to make; what's more, most are gluten free. Enjoy these main dishes with your family or cook them for yourself and have leftovers galore. There's nothing better than leftovers!

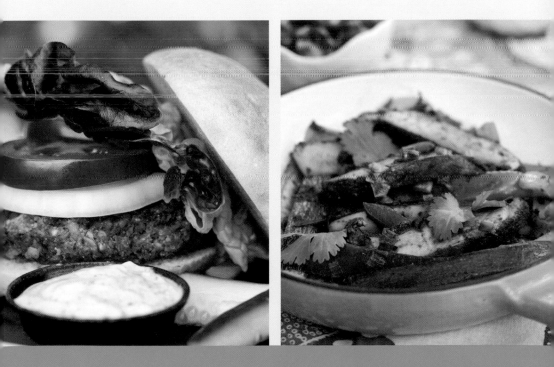

# Pasta and "Meat"balls

**6 servings**

*This recipe was inspired by my favorite vegan chef and author of Veganomincon, Isa Chandra Moskowitz. I love her spaghetti and meatballs but wanted to make a gluten-free version, so this is what I came up with. This is refined enough for grown-ups, but it even passes at the kids' table!*

Cook pasta according to package. In the meantime, puree the beans and rice in a food processor bowl until combined but some small pieces of the beans remain. Scrape into a large bowl and set aside. Add the onion, garlic, 1 tablespoon of the olive oil, Braggs, tomato paste, Worcestershire sauce, oregano, thyme, and basil. Mix well with a spoon or your hands to combine. Add the bread crumbs and mix well, using your hands, kneading until doughy. Roll into small walnut-size balls.

Heat the remaining tablespoon of olive oil in a nonstick skillet over medium heat and brown the "meatballs" on the skillet. Serve on top of spaghetti with a generous serving of marinara sauce.

1 pound gluten-free spaghetti (prepared according to package directions)

2 15-ounce cans kidney beans, drained and rinsed

½ cup cooked brown rice

½ cup yellow onion, tiny dice

2 cloves garlic, grated

2 tablespoons extra virgin olive oil

2 tablespoons Braggs Aminos

2 tablespoons tomato paste

1 tablespoon vegan Worcestershire sauce

½ teaspoon oregano

½ teaspoon thyme

¼ teaspoon basil

¼–½ cup gluten-free bread crumbs (Glutino brand is good)

1 recipe of Charlie's Tomato Sauce Marinara (page 87)

# Korean-Style Tempeh Tacos with Coleslaw

*Instead of the traditional Mexican-flavored tacos, these tacos have a Korean flair. I think you will like their savory bite, along with the crispiness of the Dijon slaw. These are really yummy served with a dollop of guacamole on top.*

Over medium heat in a large skillet, heat enough olive oil to lightly coat the bottom of the pan. Place the crumbled tempeh in the pan and cook until brown, stirring frequently. In the meantime, in a small bowl, whisk the Worcestershire sauce, tomato paste, sesame seeds, apple cider vinegar, and agave nectar. Pour over the tempeh and let it cook about 3 to 4 minutes or until the sauce is absorbed into the tempeh.

**For the slaw and dressing:** Put the cabbage, onion, and almonds in a medium-size bowl. Whisk or blend the dressing ingredients together and pour over the slaw. Stir well to combine. Season with salt and pepper.

**To assemble the tacos:** Place a spoonful of the tempeh mixture on the taco shell and top with the Dijon slaw. Add guacamole if desired.

2 tablespoons extra virgin olive oil or sesame oil

1 8-ounce package tempeh, crumbled

3 tablespoons vegan Worcestershire sauce

2 tablespoons tomato paste

2 tablespoons sesame seeds

2 tablespoons apple cider vinegar

1 tablespoon agave nectar

4–6 organic corn tortillas

## Coleslaw

½ small head red cabbage, finely shredded

¼ cup thinly sliced red onion

¼ cup sliced almonds

## Dijon Dressing

2 tablespoons Dijon mustard

1 shallot, finely diced

1 teaspoon agave nectar

4 tablespoons red wine vinegar

3 tablespoons extra virgin olive oil

Sea salt and pepper, to taste

Per Serving: Calories 210, Total Fat 11g, Saturated Fat 2g, Cholesterol 0mg, Sodium 140mg, Carbohydrate 20g, Fiber 2g, Protein 9g
Coleslaw: Calories 40, Total Fat 2g, Saturated Fat 0g, Cholesterol 0mg, Sodium 15mg, Carbohydrate 5g, Fiber 2g, Protein 2g
Dijon Dressing: Calories 70, Total Fat 7g, Saturated Fat 1g, Cholesterol 0mg, Sodium 120mg, Carbohydrate 3g, Fiber 0g, Protein 0g

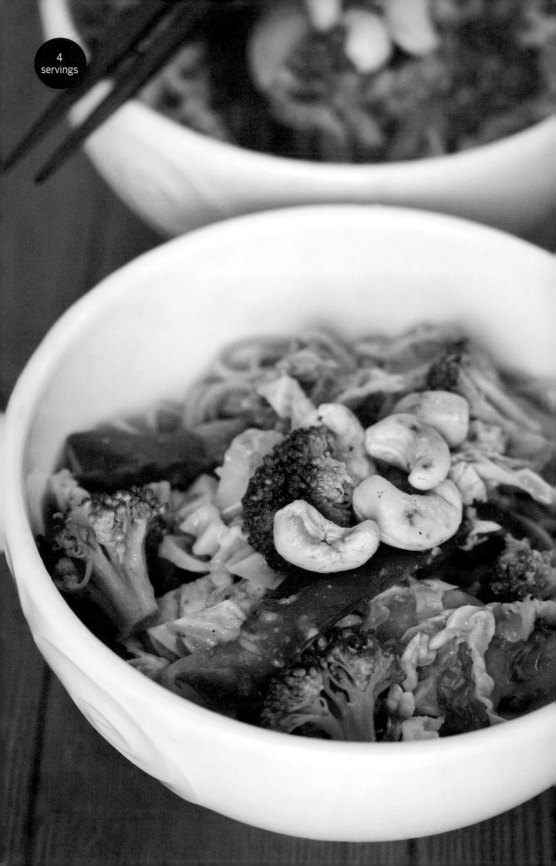

# Soba Noodle Stir-Fry
# in Creamy Cashew Sauce

*Whenever I make a stir-fry, I love to cut up the veggies
first and put them into glass bowls so I have them handy
when I start to sauté. Don't overcook the veggies;
you want them to still be crisp and bright!*

To make the sauce, blend all of the ingredients in a blender until smooth and set aside. Cook the soba noodles according to package directions. Drain and set aside.

In a large sauté pan or wok, heat the coconut oil over medium-high heat and sauté the garlic, ginger, red pepper flakes, and shallot until soft. Add the cabbage, red pepper, and broccoli, and sauté for 5 minutes until slightly soft but still crisp. Toss in the noodles, cashew sauce, and cashews and sauté for a few minutes or until sauce thickens. Serve immediately.

## Cashew Sauce

3 tablespoons cashew butter

3 tablespoons brown rice vinegar

3 tablespoons warm water

2 tablespoons Braggs Aminos

1 tablespoon agave nectar or maple syrup

1 tablespoon sesame oil

2 teaspoons arrowroot powder

## Soba Noodle Stir-Fry

10 ounces cooked buckwheat soba noodles

1 tablespoon coconut oil

2 garlic cloves, minced

1 tablespoon freshly grated ginger

½ teaspoon red pepper flakes

1 shallot, thinly sliced

1 cup shredded cabbage or bok choy

1 red bell pepper, deseeded and thinly sliced

1 cup broccoli florets

½ cup cashews, lightly toasted

Per Serving: Calories 280, Total Fat 12g, Saturated Fat 4.5g, Cholesterol 0mg, Sodium 260mg, Total Carbohydrate 36g, Fiber 4g, Protein 9g
Cashew Sauce: Calories 130, Total Fat 9g, Saturated Fat 1.5g, Cholesterol 0mg, Sodium 400mg, Carbohydrate 9g, Fiber 0g, Protein 2g

141

## Mashed Topping

3 pounds red potatoes or Yukon gold
   potatoes, cut into ½-inch cubes

⅓ cup unsweetened coconut creamer
   or unsweetened plain almond milk

1 teaspoon sea salt

2 tablespoons Earth Balance or extra
   virgin olive oil

# Un-Shepherd's Pie

*This healthier Shepherd's Pie is just as tasty as the classic comfort food. It's wonderful topped with my Savory Golden Mushroom Gravy (page 88).*

Put the potatoes in a large pot and add water, about 2 inches above the potatoes. Bring to a boil and simmer on low for about 20 minutes until very tender. Drain and put them back into the pot. Add the creamer, salt, and Earth Balance, and mash well using a potato masher or hand mixer. Set aside.

Preheat the oven to 425 degrees F and lightly grease a casserole dish with olive oil or coconut oil and set aside.

To make the filling, heat the oil in a skillet over medium heat and sauté the onion, garlic, and mushrooms until soft. Add the vinegar and cook down for a few minutes; add the celery and carrots, cooking until the carrots are tender but still a bit crisp. Stir in the tempeh and add the thyme, oregano, coriander, and Worcestershire sauce.

Dissolve the arrowroot in the broth and add to the pan with the beans. Cover and lower the heat. Cook for about 10 minutes at a simmer so the flavors meld

### Tempeh Veggie Filling

- 2 tablespoons extra virgin olive oil, plus extra for drizzling
- 1 medium yellow onion, diced
- 2 garlic cloves, minced
- 2 cups sliced mushrooms
- 2 tablespoons balsamic vinegar
- 2 stalks celery, diced
- 2 carrots, peeled and diced
- 2 8-ounce packages tempeh, crumbled
- 1 teaspoon thyme
- 1 teaspoon oregano
- 1 teaspoon coriander
- 3 tablespoons Worcestershire sauce
- 1 tablespoon arrowroot powder
- ½ cup vegetable broth
- 1 15-ounce can kidney beans, drained and rinsed
- 1 cup frozen peas
- 1 cup frozen sweet corn

and the sauce thickens. Stir occasionally so the tempeh does not stick to the pan. Remove the lid and add the peas and corn. Replace the lid and let it cook for about 2 minutes until the peas and corn are just defrosted but still crisp.

Pour the tempeh and veggie mixture into the casserole dish. Spread the mashed potato mixture on top of the veggie mixture and drizzle a little bit of olive oil on top. Bake for about 35 minutes, or until golden and bubbly. Remove from the oven and allow to cool for at least 10 minutes before serving. Scoop out into heaping servings.

Per Serving: Calories 540, Total Fat 19g, Saturated Fat 3g, Cholesterol 0mg, Sodium 1470mg, Carbohydrate 74g, Fiber 11g, Protein 26g

143

# Pad Thai in Peanut Coconut Sauce

*Pad Thai is a favorite Asian dish for many of my clients. This gluten-free version has a twist: coconut milk in the sauce, which adds depth and creaminess. You can use any type of sprouts, but mung bean sprouts are the norm. Feel free to throw in any other veggies you like, such as broccoli or edamame beans.*

## Peanut Coconut Sauce

½ cup crunchy peanut butter

3 tablespoons fresh-squeezed lime juice

1 cup coconut milk

½ teaspoon ground ginger

1 tablespoon tomato paste

2 tablespoons maple syrup

1 teaspoon red chili pepper flakes

1 teaspoon toasted sesame oil

2 tablespoons Braggs Aminos

3 tablespoons rice vinegar

## Pad Thai

12 ounces rice noodles, medium width or fettuccine style (gluten-free)

1 tablespoon sesame oil

3 garlic cloves, minced

½ medium red onion, thinly sliced

1 red bell pepper, deseeded and thinly sliced

½ cup shredded carrots

½ cup thinly cut (lengthwise) snow peas

1 cup mung bean sprouts

¼ cup crushed peanuts

5 green onions, white parts only, cut thinly lengthwise

¼ cup chopped cilantro

To make the sauce, whisk or blend all of the ingredients together until smooth. Set aside.

Cook the pasta according to the package directions. Drain and rinse with cold water.

Heat the sesame oil in a wok or large skillet over medium heat. Add the garlic and sauté for 1 minute; then add the onion, red bell pepper, carrots, and snow peas. Sauté until soft, but still crisp. Add the pasta and sauce and sauté for 3 to 4 minutes or until the sauce thickens and the dish is heated through. Remove from the heat and stir in the bean sprouts. Serve immediately and top with the crushed peanuts, green onions, and cilantro.

Per Serving: Calories 520, Total Fat 25g, Saturated Fat 10g, Cholesterol 0mg, Sodium 340mg, Total Carbohydrate 67g, Fiber 5g, Sugars 8g, Protein 11g
Peanut Coconut Sauce: Calories 520, Total Fat 25g, Saturated Fat 10g, Cholesterol 0mg, Sodium 340mg, Carbohydrate 67g, Fiber 5g, Protein 11g

# Greek Tomato Burgers

*One of my Greek clients told me about the awesome tomato "burgers" his mom used to make, so I had to come up with my own version. I made these for him, and he was transported right back to Greece and his mama's kitchen. These burgers are light, flavorful, and loaded with fiber and protein. They won't leave you feeling heavy and bogged down like an American burger can.*

Mash the beans in a food processor bowl while still maintaining some bits of bean. Scrape into a large bowl.

Heat the olive oil in a skillet over medium heat and sauté the onion and garlic until soft. Add the salt, pepper, oregano, basil, and tomatoes. Cook down until the tomatoes are mushy but still maintain their form. Add this to the mashed beans, and then add the bread crumbs, lemon juice, and flaxseed eggs. Using your hands, mash the mixture together until well combined. If the mixture is too wet, let it sit for about 10 minutes or add a touch more bread crumbs. Form into patties and brown on both sides in a skillet greased with olive oil. Serve on sprouted grain or gluten-free bread with baby greens, tomatoes, pickles, and onion.

- 2 15-ounce cans white beans or cannellini beans, drained and rinsed
- 1 tablespoon extra virgin olive oil, plus more for browning
- 1 medium yellow onion, finely diced
- 3 garlic cloves, minced
- ¾ teaspoon sea salt
- ¼ teaspoon white pepper
- 1 teaspoon dried oregano
- 1 teaspoon dried basil
- ½ cup quartered or halved cherry tomatoes
- ¾ cup gluten-free bread crumbs
- 2 teaspoons lemon juice
- 2 flaxseed eggs (page 26)

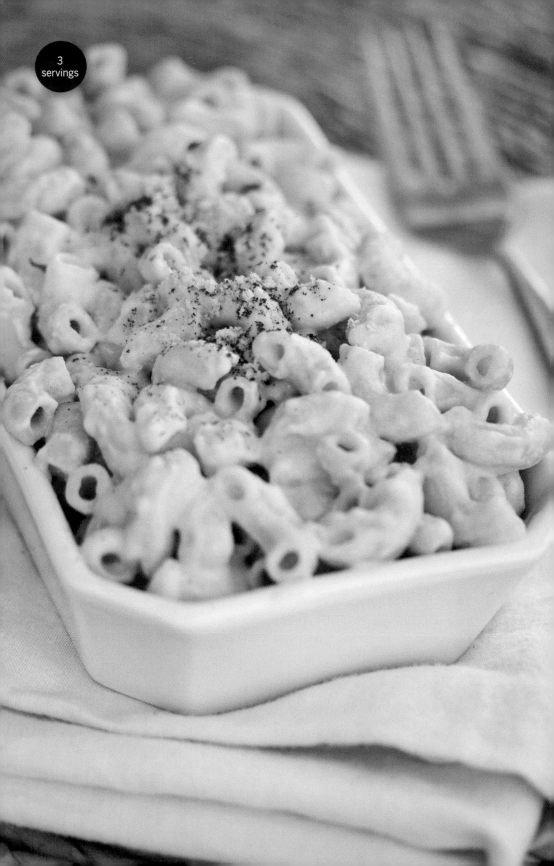

# Mac and Ch-ch-cheeeeze

*Gluten free, vegan, and oh so good! This healthier and lighter version of mac and cheese is a favorite in many kitchens. I love to add veggies like steamed broccoli or green peas to it for even more nutritional bang.*

Cook the pasta al dente. Drain and set aside. Blend the coconut milk, yeast, salt, garlic powder, onion powder, mustard, paprika, cayenne, tahini, and pepper together in a blender.

In a saucepan over medium heat, put in the olive oil and heat through. Stir in the brown rice flour and continue stirring to make a roux (a flour paste). Add the pasta and sauce mixture and cook, stirring, until the mixture boils and thickens. If the sauce is too thick, add more coconut milk; if it's too thin, add a little more rice flour. If you like a more vibrant sauce, add a touch more dry mustard and garlic or onion powder. Top with a dash of smoked paprika and serve immediately!

8 ounces gluten-free brown rice elbows or shells

1½ cups plain, unsweetened So Delicious Coconut Milk or Almond Milk

½ cup nutritional yeast

½ teaspoon sea salt

¼ teaspoon garlic powder

½ teaspoon onion powder

¼ teaspoon dry mustard

¼ teaspoon smoked paprika, plus more for garnish

Pinch cayenne pepper

1 tablespoon tahini

Pinch black pepper

2 tablespoons extra virgin olive oil or Earth Balance (soy free)

1 tablespoon brown rice flour

## Lemon Dill Aioli Dipping Sauce

1 tablespoon freshly chopped dill

¼ cup Vegenaise (grapeseed or soy free)

2 teaspoons lemon juice

1 teaspoon lemon zest

1 clove garlic, finely minced

**CHEF'S TIP**

 These fillets are also great served with my Savory Golden Mushroom Gravy (page 88).

# Chickpea Fillets

8 fillets

*These fillets are gluten-free and delicious and
great with the Lemon Dill Aioli Dipping Sauce.*

Heat 1 tablespoon of the olive oil in a skillet over medium heat. Sauté the onion, garlic, and scallions until translucent and soft. Add the thyme, marjoram, oregano, and basil. Stir to release the flavor of the herbs. Sauté for a few more minutes and then transfer to a large bowl.

In a food processor cup, combine the chickpeas and the rice. Process until well combined. Transfer to the bowl with the sautéed onions, garlic, and scallions. Add the garlic powder, onion powder, mustard powder, Braggs, the remaining tablespoon of olive oil, the bread crumbs, and the lemon zest, if using. Using your hands, mix well to combine all of the ingredients into a "dough."

2 tablespoons extra virgin olive oil or coconut oil, plus more for pan-frying

1 medium yellow onion, diced

2 garlic cloves, minced

5 scallions, white part only, thinly sliced

1 teaspoon dried thyme

½ teaspoon dried marjoram

½ teaspoon dried oregano

½ teaspoon dried basil

2 15-ounce cans chickpeas, drained and rinsed, or 3 cups cooked

1 cup cooked brown rice

½ teaspoon garlic powder

½ teaspoon onion powder

½ teaspoon dry mustard powder

1 tablespoon Braggs Aminos or soy sauce

½ cup gluten-free bread crumbs

¼ teaspoon lemon zest (optional)

Form the mixture into 8 "fillets" or patties. If baking, heat the oven to 400 degrees F, place the fillets on an oiled baking sheet, and spray with olive oil. Bake until brown (approximately 20 minutes), flipping halfway through. You can also brown the fillets in a nonstick skillet with olive oil.

To make the sauce, whisk or stir all of the ingredients together in a small bowl and serve as a dipping sauce for the fillets.

# Veggie Loaf with Tomato Glaze

*My grandmother used to make the best meat loaf in the world, made from a mixture of pork, beef, and spices. This version is plant-based and made with lentils, brown rice, and veggies, so it has a lot of fiber, protein, and nutrients. It's one of my favorites to make at holiday time, and even the meat eaters love to have a slice!*

¾ cup cooked brown rice

2 cups cooked Du Puy or French lentils

**Tomato Glaze**

1 8-ounce can tomato paste

3 tablespoons Braggs Aminos or low-sodium tamari

1 tablespoon agave nectar

¼ teaspoon liquid smoke

1 tablespoon garlic, minced

3 tablespoons extra virgin olive oil

1 cup diced onion

1 cup mushrooms, stems removed and coarsely chopped

2 stalks celery, diced

4 carrots, peeled and diced

1 tablespoon vegan Worcestershire sauce

½ teaspoon mustard powder

2 flaxseed eggs

1 tablespoon arrowroot powder

1 cup gluten-free bread crumbs

Cook the brown rice and lentils per package directions. Set aside to cool (these can also be prepared the day before and stored in the refrigerator overnight if you are short on time).

**To make the glaze:** In a small bowl, whisk together the tomato paste, 2 tablespoons of the Braggs, the agave nectar, liquid smoke, and garlic. Set aside. Preheat the oven to 350 degrees F. Grease a loaf pan with olive oil or coconut oil and set aside.

Heat 1 tablespoon of olive oil in a large skillet over medium heat and sauté the onions for approximately 5 minutes or until soft. Add the mushrooms and sauté until soft. Transfer to a small bowl.

Add the remaining 2 tablespoons of olive oil to the skillet

Per Serving: Calories 310, Total Fat 12g, Saturated Fat 2g, Cholesterol 0mg, Sodium 990mg, Total Carbohydrate 41g, Fiber 10g, Protein 11g

and sauté the celery and carrots together over low heat until semi-tender but still a bit crisp.

In a food processor, pulse the rice and lentils together until combined and somewhat smooth. Transfer to a large bowl.

In the food processor, pulse the cooked celery and carrots, Worcestershire sauce, remaining 1 tablespoon of Braggs, mustard powder, flaxseed eggs, arrowroot, and ⅓ cup of the tomato glaze until well combined. Add this mixture to the rice and lentil mixture. Fold in the sautéed onion mixture and bread crumbs. Use your hands to mix the ingredients into a doughlike consistency.

Press the mixture into the prepared loaf pan and cover with the remaining tomato glaze, spreading evenly. Cover with foil and bake for 30 minutes. Uncover and bake for an additional 15 minutes until the top is brown. Remove from the oven and cool for 15 minutes before serving.

## CHEF'S TIP

 If you cannot find Du Puy lentils, you can use regular green lentils for this dish; they are a bit mushier, so you may need extra gluten-free bread crumbs.

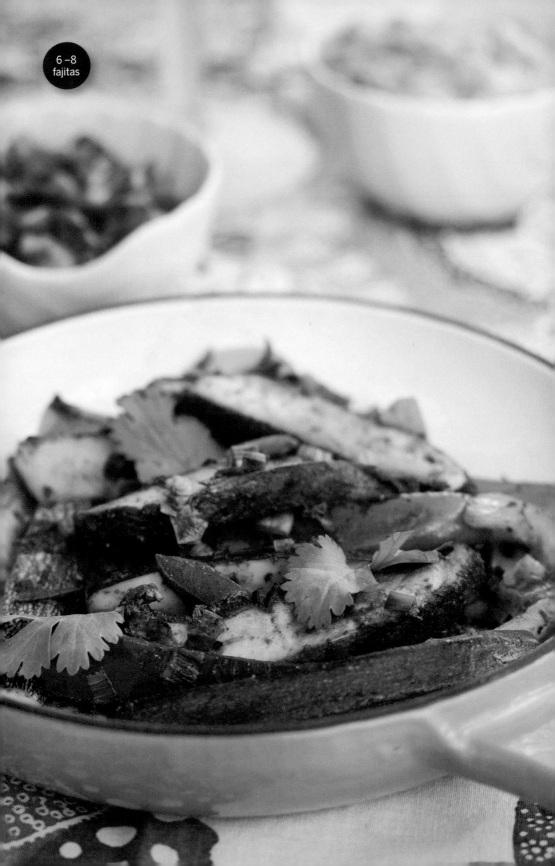

# Baja-Style Fajitas

*Fajitas are almost everyone's favorite, and these are
simple to make. I love to serve them with a side of rice and
black beans for even more flavor and nutrients.
Throw in any veggie combo you want, but I've found this
combination works the best for my taste.*

Heat the olive oil in a large skillet over medium heat and sauté the onion and mushroom. Cook for a few minutes until the onion is soft and the mushroom has released its juices. Add the bell pepper, squash, cumin, oregano, chili powder, and cilantro. Stir well to incorporate. Cover the skillet to let the veggies steam for about 5 to 7 minutes, stirring occasionally. Remove from the heat, squeeze the lime on top, and season with salt, to taste. Serve on the tortillas with a dollop of my Cashew Ricotta Cheeze (page 154) and salsa and guacamole, if preferred.

1 tablespoon extra virgin olive oil

½ large yellow onion, thinly sliced

1 large Portobello mushroom, thinly sliced

½ red bell pepper, deseeded and thinly sliced

½ green bell pepper, deseeded and thinly sliced

½ large zucchini squash, cut into ½-inch strips

1 teaspoon cumin

½ teaspoon oregano

2 teaspoons chili powder

2 tablespoons freshly chopped cilantro

Juice of one lime

Sea salt, to taste

6–8 organic yellow or blue corn soft tortillas

Salsa and guacamole (optional)

# Baked Ziti with Spinach

*This healthy version will taste just like you're eating Grandma's Italian ziti!*

2 cups Cashew Ricotta Cheeze (recipe follows)

1 pound brown rice ziti or penne, cooked al dente

1 recipe of Charlie's Tomato Sauce Marinara (page 187)

1 10-ounce bag organic, frozen chopped spinach, thawed in a colander for drainage

## Cashew Ricotta Cheeze

2 cups cashews, soaked for 4 hours

½ teaspoon onion powder

½ teaspoon garlic powder

½ teaspoon mustard powder

¼ cup nutritional yeast flakes, plus more for topping

1 teaspoon lemon juice

½ teaspoon sea salt

Filtered water

Preheat the oven to 450 degrees F. Drain the water from the cashews. Place all of the ingredients for the Cashew Ricotta Cheeze in a blender cup with just enough water to barely cover. Blend until very smooth. This mixture should be fairly thick, but if it's too thick, add more water. Pour into a bowl.

**To assemble ziti:** Pour the cooked ziti noodles into a large bowl. Ladle in the marinara sauce until well covered. Stir to coat. If you like more sauce, add more. Add 1½ cups of the Cashew Ricotta Cheeze and the thawed spinach and stir to incorporate. You can always add more cheeze if you want a "cheesier" dish. Combine with the noodles and put the mixture into a lightly oiled casserole dish. Ladle more sauce on top to cover. Sprinkle with additional nutritional yeast flakes to lightly coat. Cover with foil and bake for 30 minutes until heated through. Remove from the oven and let it cool for 5 to 10 minutes before serving.

## CHEF'S TIP

This raw vegan cheese can also be made with a combination of cashews and macadamia nuts for an even creamier texture! It's great to use as a topping for fajitas or burritos. Make an extra batch to keep in the fridge for dipping . . . or whatever.

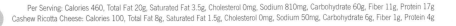
Per Serving: Calories 460, Total Fat 20g, Saturated Fat 3.5g, Cholesterol 0mg, Sodium 810mg, Carbohydrate 60g, Fiber 11g, Protein 17g
Cashew Ricotta Cheese: Calories 100, Total Fat 8g, Saturated Fat 1.5g, Cholesterol 0mg, Sodium 50mg, Carbohydrate 6g, Fiber 1g, Protein 4g

# Suprem-oh Burrito

*Who doesn't love a big fat burrito? These are great to make and freeze so you can take them on trips or in the car. If you're using gluten-free tortillas, it's best to roll them made to order, as they tend to fall apart if stored too long.*

Cook the quinoa or brown rice according to package directions and set aside. Heat the olive oil in a large skillet and sauté the peppers and onions until soft, about 5 to 7 minutes. Add the cumin, chili powder blend, and sea salt, and continue cooking for 2 more minutes, stirring to incorporate all of the spices with the peppers and onions. Add the tomatoes and stir to mix. Lower the heat and cover, cooking for about 5 to 7 minutes, until the peppers are really soft. Remove from the heat and pour into a large bowl. Add the beans and brown rice to the mixture and stir well to combine.

**To assemble burritos:** Heat the tortilla shell over a low open flame on the stove to soften or place in oven wrapped in foil at 250 degrees F until warm. Place the tortilla on a flat surface. Add 1 scoop of the pepper and onion mixture to the bottom one-third of the tortilla. Top with the Chipotle Cashew Cheeze and the avocado and salsa, if using, and roll. Serve with Chile Ranchero Sauce on top!

1 cup quinoa or brown rice

2 tablespoons extra virgin olive oil

1 red bell pepper, deseeded and sliced into thin strips

1 yellow bell pepper, deseeded and sliced into thin strips

1 medium red onion, thinly sliced into half moons

2 teaspoons ground cumin

1 tablespoon chili powder blend

½ teaspoon sea salt

1 15-ounce can fire roasted or regular diced tomatoes

1 15-ounce can organic black beans

1 package (6) gluten-free or sprouted grain tortillas

¼ cup Chipotle Cashew Cheeze Sauce (page 85)

Avocado and salsa (optional)

½ cup Chile Ranchero Sauce (page 89)

Per Serving: Calories 410, Total Fat 12g, Saturated Fat 1g, Cholesterol 0mg, Sodium 700mg, Carbohydrate 60g, Fiber 11g, Protein 15g

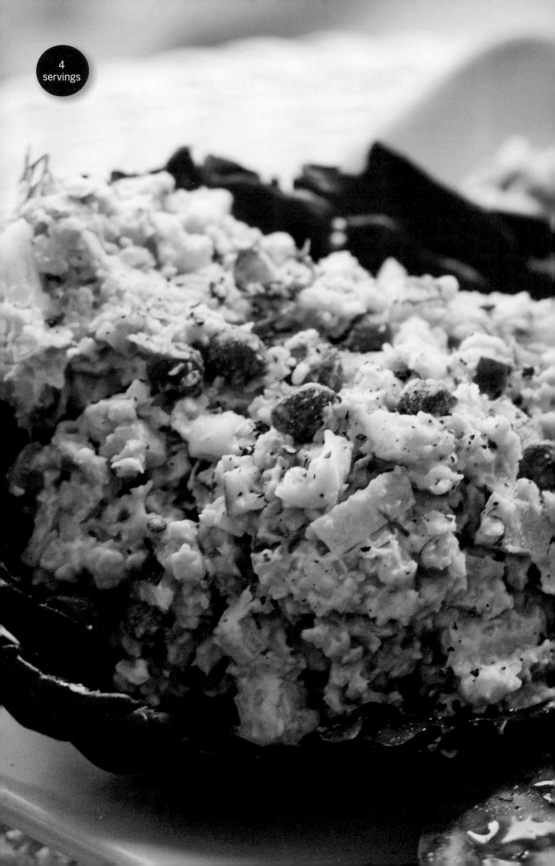

# Chickpea "Tuna" Salad

*You really won't miss the tuna in this vegan version of tuna salad. It's made with chickpeas, which, when ground in a food processor to a flaky consistency, kind of resemble our finned friend. If you can't find grapeseed Vegenaise (such as Follow Your Heart brand), any vegan mayo will be fine. I love to serve this on a bed of greens or roll it up in a gluten-free tortilla with some lettuce.*

Using a food processor fitted with the S-blade, grind the chickpeas to small flaky pieces. Add to a bowl with the remaining ingredients and mix well using a large spoon. Season with salt and pepper.

2 15-ounce cans chickpeas, drained and rinsed

1 small red onion, diced

3 scallions, thinly sliced

2 tablespoons capers

1 tablespoon fresh chopped dill or 1 teaspoon dried

¼ cup chopped walnuts or sliced almonds

3 tablespoons grapeseed Vegenaise

1 tablespoon Dijon mustard

2 teaspoons apple cider vinegar

Sea salt and pepper, to taste

# Curried Tempeh Salad

*This is a great salad to serve on a bed of lettuce as
an entrée at lunch. It's packed with protein, fiber, and flavor.
It's also one of my favorites to take on a picnic or to
use to make tea sandwiches for a party.*

1 8-ounce package tempeh, diced into ¼-inch cubes

1 15-ounce can chickpeas

2 celery stalks, diced

½ small red onion, diced

1 green apple, diced

2 tablespoons chopped dried cranberries or currants

2 teaspoons curry powder

½ teaspoon sea salt

2 tablespoons rice wine vinegar

2 tablespoons Vegenaise (Follow Your Heart brand is best) or any vegan mayonnaise

Steam the tempeh for 7 to 8 minutes in a steamer basket or in a small amount of water in a pot with a tight-fitting lid. Mash the chickpeas with a fork or food processor. Put into a large mixing bowl. Remove the tempeh from the stove and let cool. Once cool, add it to the chickpeas. Combine with the remaining ingredients and stir well to incorporate all of the flavors.

**CHEF'S TIP**

Steaming tempeh helps to get rid of some of the bitterness it can have when uncooked.

Per Serving: Calories 330, Total Fat 13g, Saturated Fat 2.5g, Cholesterol 0mg, Sodium 360mg, Carbohydrate 37g, Fiber 8g, Protein 18g

# Fresh Pesto, Tomato, and Zucchini Pasta

In a skillet, heat the olive oil over medium heat. Add the garlic and onion. Cook until translucent. Add the zucchini, mushrooms, oregano, and dried thyme and cook until slightly brown. Add the Roma tomatoes and the canned tomatoes and cover for about 5 minutes so that the tomatoes reduce down.

**To make the pesto:** Combine the cilantro, pine nuts, and garlic in a food processor and blend until the ingredients begin forming a paste. Scrape the sides of the bowl as necessary. Add the lemon juice and blend more. While the motor is running, drizzle in the olive oil, along with the salt and pepper, and process until smooth and creamy. Add additional oil if necessary.

Add the pesto to the zucchini mixture and stir to combine. Serve immediately over the pasta.

2 tablespoons olive oil

3 cloves garlic, diced

1 medium red onion, diced

1 pound brown rice fusilli pasta, cooked according to package instructions

2 medium zucchini, cut into quarters and diced

1 cup chopped mushrooms

1 teaspoon dried oregano

1 teaspoon dried thyme

4 Roma tomatoes, diced

1 15-ounce can fire-roasted diced tomatoes

¼ cup Cilantro Pesto (recipe follows)

## Cilantro Pesto

2 large bunches of cilantro, stems removed (about 3 cups, loosely packed)

¼ cup pine nuts

2–3 whole garlic cloves

½ lemon, juiced

3 tablespoons extra virgin olive oil

Sea salt and pepper, to taste

Per Serving: Calories 600, Total Fat 14g, Saturated Fat 1.5g, Cholesterol 0mg, Sodium 280mg, Carbohydrate 101g, Fiber 14g, Protein 18g
Cilantro Pesto: Per Serving: Calories 170, Total Fat 17g, Saturated Fat 2g, Cholesterol 0mg, Sodium 20mg, Carbohydrate 4g, Fiber 2g, Protein 2g

# Quinoa and Currant Stuffed Bell Peppers

8 servings

*These are the perfect mix of spicy and sweet. They make a great meal when served with a large, leafy green salad. This is also an awesome dish to take to a small dinner party or potluck.*

Preheat the oven to 350 degrees F. Fill a baking dish with about 1 inch of water. Heat the olive oil in a saucepan over medium heat. Add the onion, celery, and garlic, and cook about 5 minutes or until soft. Add the cumin, coriander, and cayenne, and stir to combine and release the flavor of the spices. Stir in the spinach and let it wilt. Add the tomatoes and salt. Cook for about 5 minutes or until most of the liquid has evaporated. Stir in the black beans, currants, nutritional yeast, quinoa, and 2 cups of water. Bring to a boil and then reduce the heat to medium low; cover and simmer for 20 minutes or until the quinoa is tender.

Fill each half pepper with about three-quarters cup of the quinoa mixture and place in the baking dish. Cover with foil and bake for one hour. Uncover and bake about 10 minutes more, or until the tops of the stuffed peppers are browned. Remove from the oven and let the peppers sit for 5 minutes before serving.

2 tablespoons extra virgin olive oil

1 medium yellow onion, diced

2 celery stalks, diced

2 cloves garlic, minced

2 teaspoons cumin

1 teaspoon coriander

¼ teaspoon cayenne pepper

2 cups chopped baby spinach

1 28-ounce can fire-roasted diced tomatoes

1 teaspoon sea salt

1 15-ounce can black beans

¼ cup currants

2 tablespoons nutritional yeast

¾ cup quinoa

2 cups water

4 large yellow or red bell peppers, cut in half lengthwise and deseeded

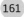

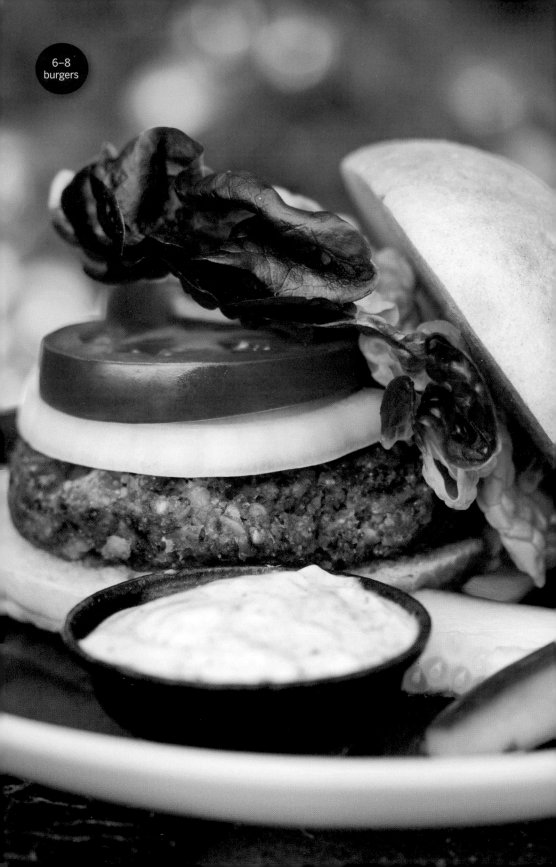

# Karma Burgers with Chipotle Mayo

*These veggie burgers are the biggest hit with my clients.
I make them by the dozen for their freezers! I love to eat one on a
sprouted grain roll with a dollop of Chipotle Mayo (recipe below),
pickles, agave ketchup, and avocado. Double the batch and wrap them
individually for your freezer. These babies are good karma!*

Using a food processor, puree the pepper, onion, spinach, and cilantro until well combined into a liquid. Scrape into a medium-size bowl. In a food processor, puree the brown rice and chickpeas together into a paste, then add to the bowl containing the veggie mixture. Add the chili powder, tomato paste, and salt. Stir together to mix well (I love to use my hands to make sure all the ingredients are combined really well). Add the bread crumbs and combine until mixture sticks together. If the burgers feel too wet, add a touch more bread crumbs. Form into patties and cook on a skillet with olive oil over medium heat until browned on both sides.

**For the Chipotle Mayo:**
Stir the ingredients together in a small bowl.

½ red bell pepper, deseeded and cut into chunks

½ medium red or yellow onion, cut into chunks

2 cups baby spinach leaves

½ bunch cilantro

¾ cup cooked brown rice

1 13-ounce can chickpeas, drained and rinsed

1 teaspoon chili powder

2 tablespoons tomato paste

½ teaspoon sea salt

1½–2 cups gluten-free bread crumbs

Extra virgin olive oil for browning

## Chipotle Mayo (¼ cup)

¼ cup grapeseed Vegenaise (such as Follow Your Heart)

¼ teaspoon chipotle chili powder

½ teaspoon agave nectar

Per Serving: Calories 150, Total Fat 5g, Saturated Fat 1g, Cholesterol 0mg, Sodium 520mg, Carbohydrate 20g, Fiber 4g, Protein 6g
Chipotle Mayo: Per Serving: Calories 90, Total Fat 9g, Saturated Fat 1.5g, Cholesterol 0mg, Sodium 85mg, Carbohydrate 2g, Fiber 0g, Protein 0g

# Cha-Cha Enchiladarole

*This dish is an enchilada casserole, or an enchiladarole,
which I know will be one of your favorites. Feel free to freeze half
if you can't finish the whole tray in one sitting. The combination of
the Chipotle Cashew Cheeze Sauce (page 85), corn tortillas, and
Chile Ranchero Sauce (page 89) will transport you right to Mexico!*

1 medium yellow onion, diced

1 green bell pepper, deseeded and diced

2 garlic cloves, minced

1 tablespoon extra virgin olive oil

1 8-ounce package tempeh, crumbled

2 teaspoons cumin

1 teaspoon chili powder

2 tablespoons nutritional yeast, plus more for dusting

1 tablespoon Braggs Aminos or low-sodium tamari

1½ cups diced Roma tomatoes

2 teaspoons lime juice

¼ cup water

1 large garnet yam, peeled and cut into ¼-inch cubes

2 15-ounce cans black beans, drained and rinsed

1 package (12) organic soft corn tortillas

3 cups Chile Ranchero Sauce (page 89)

1½ cups Chipotle Cashew Cheeze Sauce (page 85)

Preheat the oven to 350 degrees F. In a large skillet over medium heat, sauté the onion, green pepper, and garlic in olive oil until soft. Add the tempeh, cumin, chili powder, nutritional yeast, and Braggs. Stir to combine well and cook for about 2 to 3 minutes. Add the tomatoes, lime juice, water, and yam. Cover with a lid, and cook about 15 minutes until the yam is soft and the liquid is reduced. Uncover and add the black beans. Stir to combine and cook for approximately 2 more minutes, or until the beans are heated through.

Per Serving: Calories 610, Total Fat 22g, Saturated Fat 4g, Cholesterol 0mg, Sodium 1030mg, Carbohydrate 79g, Fiber 20g, Protein 31g

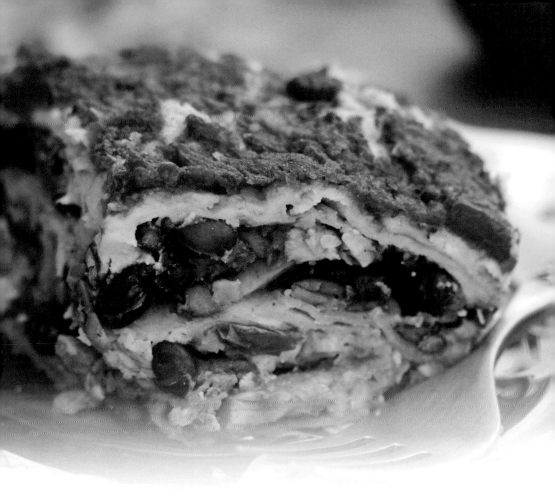

**To assemble casserole:** Ladle the Chile Ranchero Sauce in a thin layer on the bottom of a casserole dish. Line with four to six corn tortillas. Pour the tempeh mixture on top of the tortillas. Scoop ¾ cup of Chipotle Cashew Cheeze Sauce and spread it evenly over the mixture using a spatula or large spoon. Top with another couple of ladles of Chile Ranchero Sauce to make a thin layer. Finish off with one last layer of tortillas and top with Ranchero Sauce. Sprinkle the nutritional yeast on top in a light dusting. Bake in the oven, uncovered, for approximately 10 minutes or until bubbly and starting to brown. Let it sit for about 10 minutes uncovered and then cut and serve.

## CHEF'S TIP

 Short on time? Buy premade ranchero sauce at the grocery store, but watch out for added sugars.

# Chapter 6

## *Simply Sublime Sides*

When I go to a non-vegan restaurant, I often find myself ordering from the side dish menu. I find that I can make a nutritious meal out of three different side dishes. I love to make sides at home and serve them with a bed of grains or a leafy green salad for a healthy, well-rounded meal loaded with nutrients and a variety of flavors. Almost all of these dishes are a snap to make, so you can easily throw together a few and chow down in a healthified eating frenzy!

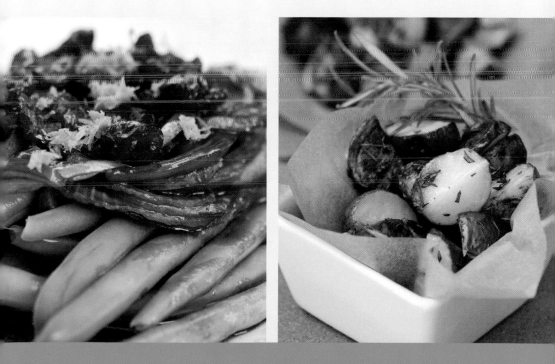

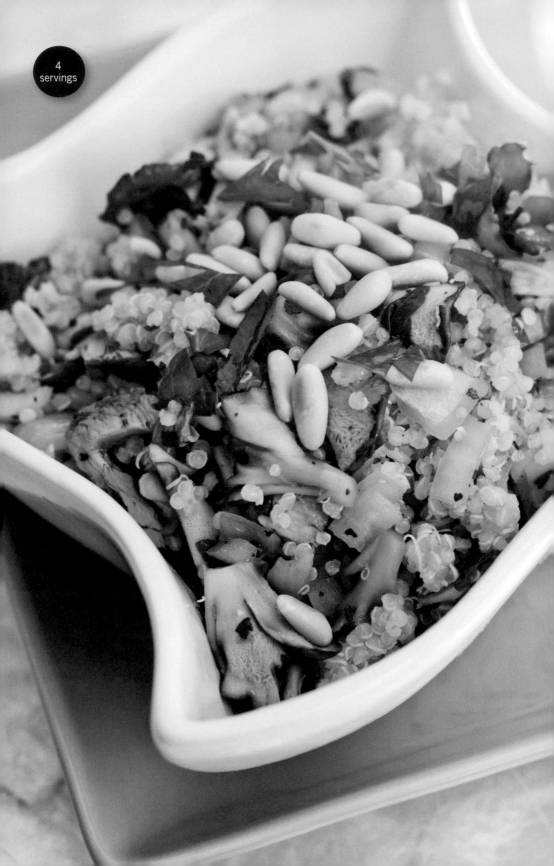

# Wild Mushroom Quinoa Pilaf

*Quinoa is so packed with protein that I wanted to use it
in this dish instead of the normal pilaf ingredient of rice. It's nutty,
light, and it cooks easily. Use any combination of mushrooms you
can find. This dish is earthy, woody, and superdelicious.*

Put the cooked quinoa in a large bowl and set aside. Heat the olive oil in a large skillet over medium heat and sauté the garlic and onion until soft. Add the mushrooms and vinegar and season with salt and pepper to your liking. Cook until the mushrooms are soft and releasing their juices, about 5 minutes. Add the parsley, oregano, and pine nuts. Pour over the quinoa and add the lemon juice. Toss to combine.

1 cup cooked quinoa

1 tablespoon extra virgin olive oil

2 cloves garlic, minced

½ medium onion, finely diced

2 cups variety of wild mushrooms (oyster, shiitake, morels, and/or Portobello)

1 tablespoon red wine vinegar

Sea salt and ground pepper, to taste

2 tablespoons fresh chopped parsley

1 teaspoon dried oregano

¼ cup lightly toasted pine nuts, for serving

Juice from ½ lemon

Per Serving: Calories 160, Total Fat 10g, Saturated Fat 1g, Cholesterol 0mg, Sodium 5mg, Carbohydrate 14g, Fiber 3g, Protein 5g

169

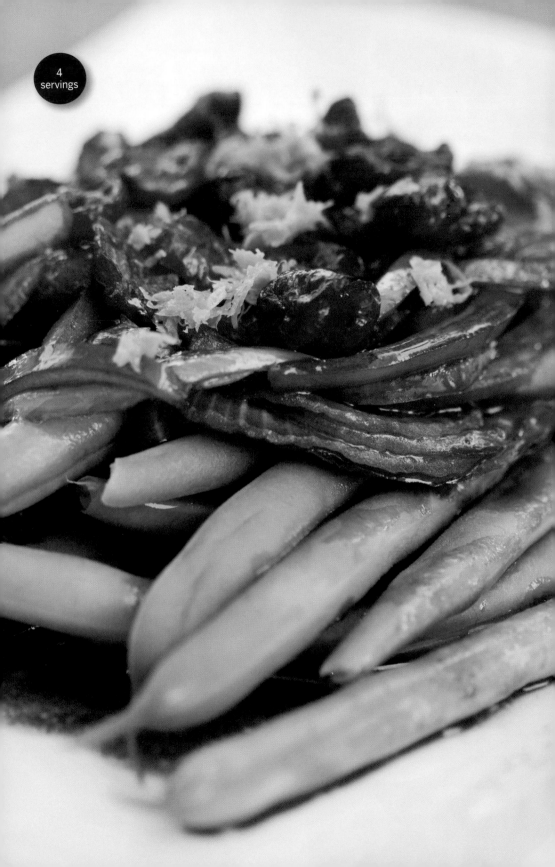

4
servings

# Cranberry Balsamic Green Beans

*There is nothing like crisp green beans served on
the side of a beautiful and delicious main dish. These are
tangy and sweet at the same time. I like to buy bags of cranberries
at holiday time when they are more readily available and
keep them in my freezer for use all year round.*

Steam or blanch the green beans until fork tender, 5 to 15 minutes depending on the size of the beans. Drain and set aside. In a large skillet, melt the coconut oil over medium heat. Add the onions and sauté until translucent. Turn up the heat slightly and caramelize the onions until golden, stirring occasionally, about 10 minutes. Add the cranberries, orange zest, orange juice, vinegar, and pomegranate, or cherry juice. Simmer until the liquid is reduced by about half. Add the green beans and toss to coat. Serve immediately.

2 pounds fresh green beans, trimmed

1–2 tablespoons coconut oil

1 medium red onion, thinly sliced

¼ cup dried cranberries

Zest and juice from 1 medium orange

2 tablespoons balsamic vinegar

3 tablespoons pomegranate juice or cherry juice (not from concentrate)

Per Serving: Calories 150, Total Fat 6g, Saturated Fat 4.5g, Cholesterol 0mg, Sodium 15mg, Carbohydrate 25g, Fiber 7g, Protein 4g

171

# Norwegian Sweet and Sour Cabbage

*Every Christmas Eve, my Norwegian sister-in-law, Ingvild, makes this amazing sweet-and-sour cabbage. I told her I must have the recipe for my cookbook, and she obliged. I cleaned it up a bit and got rid of the processed sugar and added maple syrup instead. You are welcome to use maple syrup if you want an earthier flavor.*

1 tablespoon coconut oil

½ red large onion, thinly sliced

1 large head of red cabbage, shredded

½ large head white cabbage, shredded

3 apples, cored and diced (a Granny Smith and Fuji combo is really good)

1½ cups vegetable broth

¼ teaspoon cloves

3 tablespoons apple cider vinegar

2 tablespoons maple syrup

1 teaspoon sea salt

¼ cup dried cranberries (optional)

Heat the coconut oil over medium heat and add the onion, sautéing until soft. Add the remaining ingredients to the pot except the cranberries. Stir well to combine, cover, and simmer for approximately 30 minutes, stirring occasionally until the cabbage and apples are soft. Top with cranberries before serving.

Per Serving: Calories 140, Total Fat 2g, Saturated Fat 1.5g, Cholesterol 0mg, Sodium 420mg, Carbohydrate 31g, Fiber 6g, Protein 3g

# Apple Cherry Chutney

**About 3½ cups**

*Tangy, sweet, and sour flavors combine in this delicious chutney, which is fabulous served with Mashed Coconut Yams with Cardamom (page 183). It's also great to use as a spread on sandwiches or on crackers with a dollop of Chipotle Cashew Cheeze Sauce (page 85).*

Place all of the ingredients into a saucepan over medium heat. Bring to a boil and then lower the heat and simmer until all of the ingredients are soft, the liquid is evaporated, and the chutney thickens. Stir occasionally to prevent burning. Remove from the heat and cool. Serve chilled. Store in a container with a tight-fitting lid for up to two weeks.

1 cup dried cherries

3 apples, cored and chopped into small pieces (1 Granny Smith plus 2 Golden Delicious)

¼ cup chopped dried apricots

¼ cup raisins or currants (optional)

2 tablespoons apple cider vinegar

1 cup apple cider or fresh orange juice

¼ cup water

½ cup agave nectar or maple syrup

1½ tablespoons freshly grated ginger

1 teaspoon ground cinnamon

1 cinnamon stick

Pinch cloves

¼ teaspoon sea salt

Zest of one orange (optional)

Per Serving: Calories 30, Total Fat 0g, Saturated Fat 0g, Cholesterol 0mg, Sodium 15mg, Carbohydrate 8g, Fiber 1g, Protein 0g

173

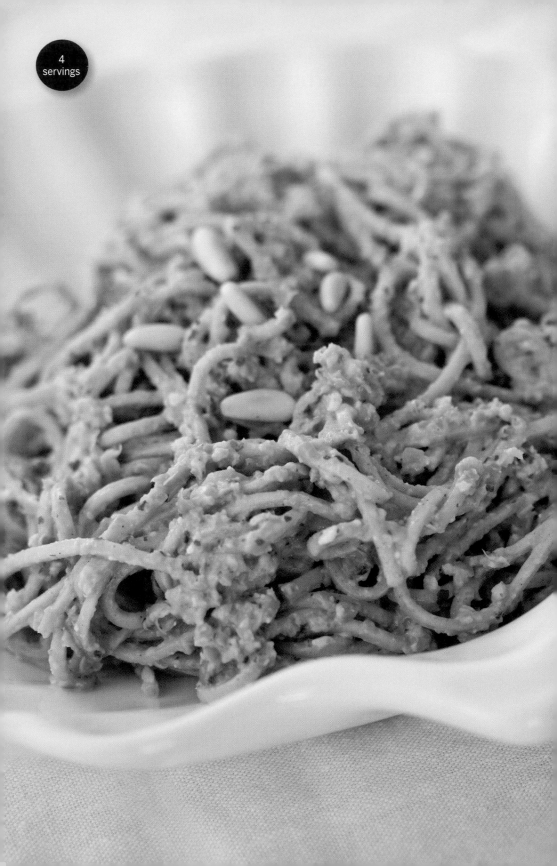

# Soba Noodle and Pea Pesto

*Amazing natural food chef Agi G of One More Bite
created this beautiful and simple side dish, which uses sweet peas
instead of basil for pesto. You can serve this dish chilled or
slightly warmed; either way it's brilliant and delicious!*

Cook the soba noodles according to the package directions, drain, and set aside in a large bowl. Combine the peas, garlic, pine nuts, and mint in a food processor and pulse a couple of times until all are roughly combined. Add the salt and pepper to taste and then the lemon zest, and close the lid again. With the processor running, slowly pour the olive oil into the mixture until creamy and well combined. Scoop the pesto over the noodles and gently mix together using tongs. Sprinkle with additional pine nuts before serving.

- 1 8.8-ounce package of soba noodles (gluten-free buckwheat is best)
- 1 10-ounce bag of frozen sweet peas, thawed
- 2 garlic cloves
- ½ cup toasted pine nuts, plus a few extra for garnish
- ½ cup fresh mint, plus a few extra leaves for garnish
- Sea salt and pepper, to taste
- 1 tablespoon lemon zest
- ⅓ cup extra virgin olive oil

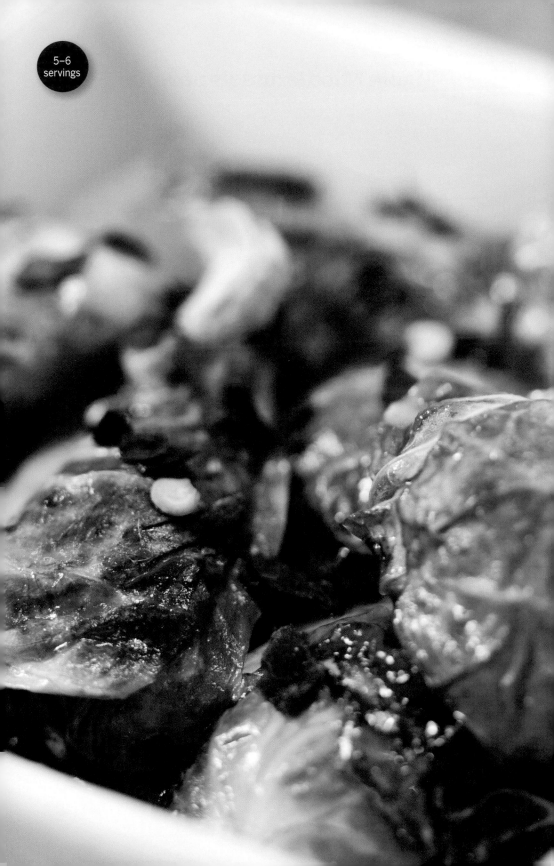

5–6
servings

# Maple Miso Brussels Sprouts

*This side dish is sweet, salty, and so delicious.*
*Brussels sprouts are usually not a favorite in many households,*
*but I think you will become a convert after eating these.*
*They are great to serve at a holiday dinner table or anytime, really!*

Preheat the oven to 400 degrees F. Place the Brussels sprouts in a large bowl. Blend together the remaining ingredients (including the pepper) in a blender until smooth. Pour the mixture over the sprouts and toss to coat. Spread the sprouts onto a large baking sheet lined with parchment paper. Roast for about 40 minutes, making sure to stir the sprouts a few times during roasting to even out the browning.

3 pounds Brussels sprouts, ends trimmed off and cut into halves

3 tablespoons extra virgin olive oil

2 tablespoons mellow white miso

2 tablespoons maple syrup

1 tablespoon Braggs Aminos or low-sodium tamari

½ cup toasted, chopped hazelnuts

Freshly ground pepper, to taste

# Chili Sweet Potato Batons

*Sweet potato "fries" without all the guilt.*
*Sweet and spicy, these batons go great with a sandwich*
*at lunch or as a hearty side dish at dinner. Loaded with*
*complex carbs and fiber, these will satisfy you*
*without the heaviness of fried potatoes.*

2 large garnet yams, peeled and cut into
½-inch-thick lengthwise batons

2–4 tablespoons extra virgin olive oil

3 teaspoons chili powder blend

Sea salt, to taste

Preheat the oven to 400 degrees F. Place the cut potatoes in a large bowl and drizzle with olive oil to coat. Season with the chili powder blend and salt. Using your hands (or a large spoon if you prefer), toss the potatoes around to evenly coat with the seasoning. Spread the potatoes in a single layer on a baking tray lined with parchment paper. Bake in the oven for about 20 to 30 minutes, turning occasionally until browned and tender. Let them cool for 5 minutes before serving.

Per Serving: Calories 210, Total Fat 14g, Saturated Fat 2g, Cholesterol 0mg, Sodium 90mg, Carbohydrate 19g, Fiber 4g, Protein 2g

# Spaghetti Squash Italiano

*Spaghetti squash is so awesome because it's a healthy alternative to regular processed, high-carb spaghetti. I love this Italian version, but sometimes I make it with Indian spices, such as cardamom and cumin, for a different flavor altogether. Get creative and experiment!*

Preheat the oven to 375 degrees F. Cut the squash in half lengthwise and remove the seeds. Place the squash in a large baking dish, cut side down. Add about ½ inch of water to the dish. Bake for about 40 minutes or until the squash is fork tender. Remove from the oven and let it cool slightly. Using a fork, scrape out spaghetti-like strands and discard the skins. Set the squash aside.

In the meantime, heat the olive oil in a skillet and sauté the garlic and red onion with the red pepper flakes until the onions are soft and slightly caramelized. Add the mushrooms, zucchini, oregano, basil, and vinegar. Stir to combine and cook for about 5 minutes or until the mushrooms cook down and the zucchini softens. Add the tomatoes, nutritional yeast, salt, and pepper, and cook for about 7 more minutes to let the tomatoes simmer and meld with the other flavors. Serve over the top of the warm spaghetti squash.

- 1 4-pound spaghetti squash
- 1 tablespoon extra virgin olive oil
- 2 garlic cloves, minced
- 1 cup finely chopped red onion
- ¼ teaspoon crushed red pepper flakes
- ½ cup finely chopped baby Portobello mushrooms
- 1 cup chopped zucchini
- 2 teaspoons dried oregano
- 1 teaspoon dried basil
- 2 teaspoons red wine vinegar
- 1 28-ounce can of fire-roasted diced tomatoes
- 2 tablespoons nutritional yeast
- ½ teaspoon sea salt
- Freshly ground black pepper

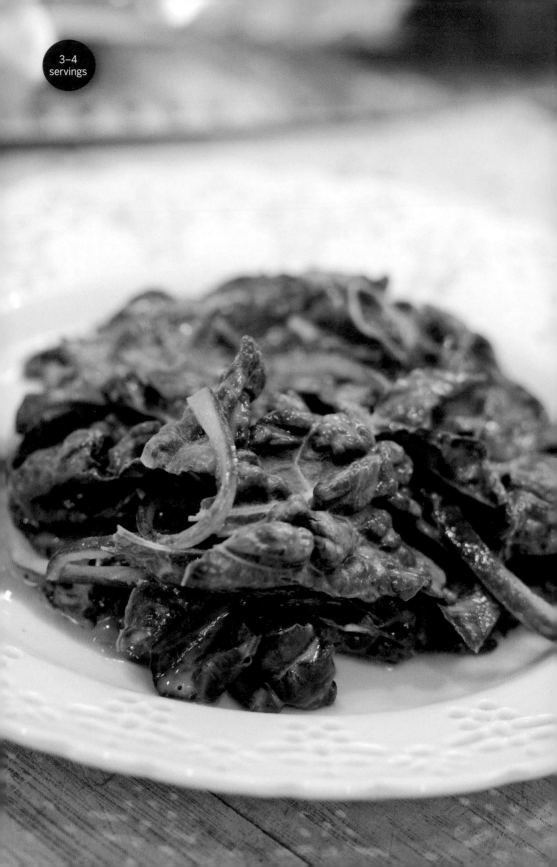

3–4
servings

# Creamy Tahini Kale

*Kale is one of my favorite greens to eat.
My body actually craves it now. This deliciously creamy
tahini sauce gives kale a whole new life. Creamy, savory,
and tangy, this side dish will liven up any meal!*

Blend all of the sauce ingredients together in a blender until smooth. Set aside.

Heat the coconut oil in a skillet over medium heat and sauté the shallots until translucent and starting to brown. Add the kale and the tahini sauce. Cover and steam for 5 minutes, stirring occasionally until the sauce begins to thicken. Garnish with sesame seeds, if desired, before serving.

### Tahini Sauce

⅓ cup tahini

2 tablespoons balsamic vinegar or Umeboshi vinegar

3 tablespoons tamari

1 cup filtered water

1 tablespoon coconut oil or extra virgin olive oil

2 shallots, diced

1 bunch kale, stems removed and ripped into large pieces

Sesame seeds (optional for garnish)

Per Serving: Calories 230, Total Fat 15g, Saturated Fat 4.5g, Cholesterol 0mg, Sodium 820mg, Total Carbohydrate 21g, Fiber 4g, Protein 9g

181

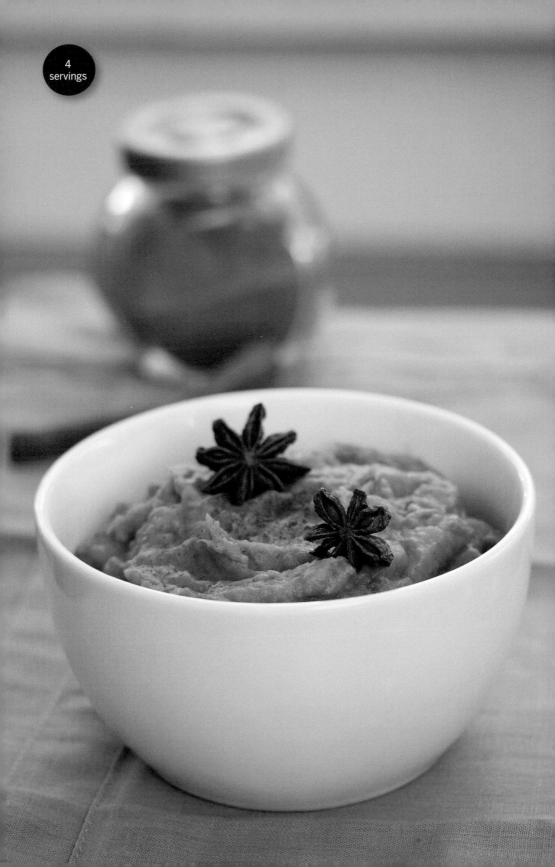

# Mashed Coconut Yams
# with Cardamom

*This is one of my favorite holiday side dishes.*
*My mom always made candied yams for the holidays,*
*which were loaded with sugar and butter and oh so good,*
*but this dish is much healthier and just as tasty.*
*I love the creaminess of yams when you mash them up.*
*It's like eating candy!*

Preheat the oven to 400 degrees F. Scrub the skins of the yams and dry. Poke multiple holes in the yams with a fork and place them on a baking sheet lined with parchment paper. Bake for about 30 minutes or until they are soft all the way through. Remove from the oven. Let them cool slightly and then carefully remove the skin and scoop the flesh out into a bowl. Add the coconut milk, cardamom, and salt, and mash them together using a fork or spoon. Serve immediately.

3 large garnet yams

1 cup full-fat canned coconut milk

½ teaspoon cardamom

½ teaspoon salt

4
servings

# Blissed-Out Herb-Roasted Taters

*Simple, nutritious, and herbalicious!*
*There is nothing that says comfort more than roasted*
*potatoes, which are healthier than their fried counterparts.*
*Eat these beauties served with my Chipotle Cashew Cheeze Sauce*
*(page 85) drizzled on top, and you will be in heaven!*

Preheat the oven to 400 degrees F. Toss the potatoes in the olive oil with the fresh herbs and the salt to taste. Spread evenly on a baking sheet lined with parchment paper and bake for 30 to 40 minutes or until soft and the edges start to turn brown. Turn the potatoes once or twice while baking.

2 pounds baby red potatoes, cut in halves

3 tablespoons extra virgin olive oil

2 tablespoons freshly chopped rosemary

2 tablespoons freshly chopped thyme

Sea salt, to taste

 **Karmic Health Tip:** *Red potatoes or red bliss potatoes contain the lowest amount of sugar of any potato, so they won't spike your blood sugar like their white amigos! Leave the skins on for extra fiber and nutrients.*

Per Serving: Calories 260, Total Fat 11g, Saturated Fat 1.5g, Cholesterol 0mg, Sodium 40mg, Carbohydrate 37g, Fiber 4g, Protein 4g

# Cilantro Cauliflower Smash

*This is an awesome alternative to high-glycemic
and high-fat mashed potatoes. These are loaded with fiber,
flavor, and tons of nutrition. I guarantee you won't
look back for those white spuds ever again.*

3 tablespoons extra virgin olive oil

2 medium fresh leeks, white parts
 only, thinly sliced

1 medium head of cauliflower,
 cut into florets

Handful fresh cilantro

2 15-ounce cans white beans,
 drained and rinsed

¼ cup unsweetened coconut
 creamer or unsweetened
 nondairy milk

1 teaspoon sea salt

Heat 1 tablespoon of olive oil in a large frying pan over medium-high heat and sauté the leeks until soft and golden brown. In the meantime, steam the cauliflower in a steamer basket (or a pot with a lid) until tender, 5 to 7 minutes or so. Set aside and cool a bit. Combine the sautéed leeks, cauliflower, cilantro, and beans in a food processor and puree until smooth. Add the coconut creamer, the 2 remaining tablespoons of olive oil, and the salt, and puree again until smooth. Scrape down the sides of the processor cup as needed. Serve warm.

Per Serving: Calories 200, Total Fat 6g, Saturated Fat 1g, Cholesterol 0mg, Sodium 330mg, Carbohydrate 29g, Fiber 7g, Protein 10g

# Hurried Curried Greens

*Leafy greens are so good for us, but most people don't know how to make them taste good. I think you will enjoy this tangy and spicy side dish. I love to serve these greens over a bed of quinoa or rice with a side salad for a light meal.*

Heat the coconut oil in a large skillet over medium heat and sauté the shallots until dark brown and caramelized, approximately 20 minutes. In the meantime, whisk together the remaining ingredients in a bowl. Add the greens to the sauté pan and pour the sauce on top. Cover and steam for 5 minutes, stirring occasionally, until the greens are still chewy but tender.

1 tablespoon coconut oil

2 shallots, diced

1 tablespoon curry powder

1 tablespoon agave nectar

2 tablespoons low-sodium tamari or Braggs Aminos

1 tablespoon water

2 teaspoons fresh lemon juice

1 bunch leafy greens, stripped of stems and ripped into large pieces (Swiss chard, collard greens, kale, or any other leafy greens available)

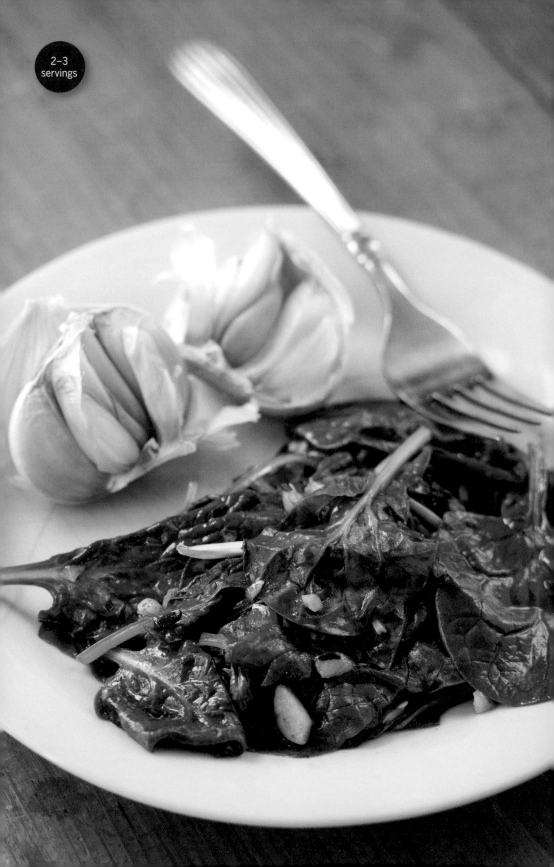

2–3
servings

# Spicy Garlic Spinach

*Garlic and spinach are two of my favorite ingredients.
This is reminiscent of my father's Italian cooking, and it's so simple
to make. It's one of my go-to side dishes in a pinch to
add extra iron and nutrients to my meal.*

In a sauté pan, heat the olive oil over medium heat. Add the garlic and red pepper flakes and sauté until soft. Add the spinach. Cover and let the spinach wilt. Serve immediately.

1 tablespoon extra virgin olive oil

3 garlic cloves, minced

½ teaspoon red pepper flakes

1 large bunch fresh spinach, washed well

Per Serving: Calories 80, Total Fat 5g, Saturated Fat 1g, Cholesterol 0mg, Sodium 120mg, Carbohydrate 7g, Fiber 3g, Protein 5g

189

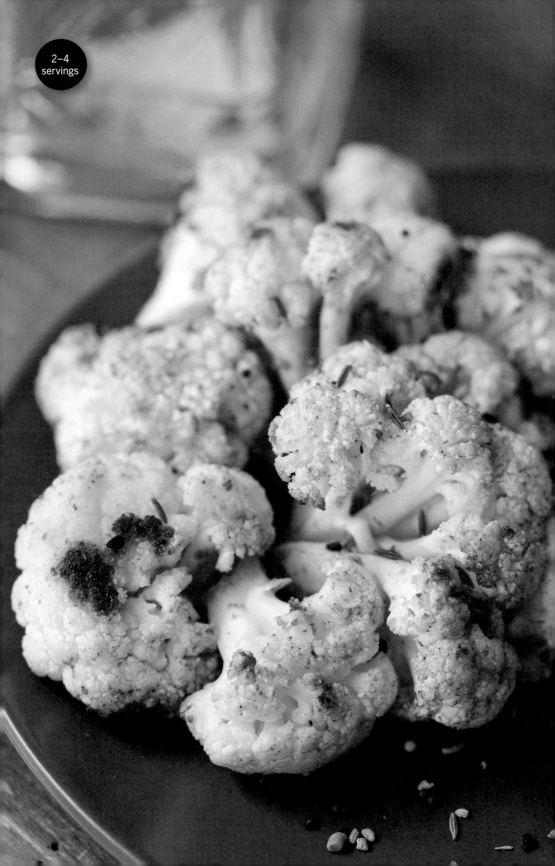

2–4
servings

# Cumin Cauliflower Roast

*This savory side dish is great served with
grains and a large leafy green salad. I also love to eat
it alone as a healthy afternoon snack.*

Preheat the oven to 350 degrees F. Toss the cauliflower in a bowl with the cumin, olive oil, and sea salt to taste. Spread in a single layer onto a baking sheet lined with parchment paper and roast until tender and slightly brown, about 20 minutes.

1 large head of cauliflower, cut into bite-size pieces

2 teaspoons cumin

3 tablespoons extra virgin olive oil

Sea salt, to taste

# Chapter 7

# Ooey, Gooey, and Delightfully Decadent Desserts

*I* *love dessert, and because of this sweet tooth,* I have spent many years finding ways to make desserts healthier yet still tasty. You won't find any white sugar or flour here, but you will find lots of taste, texture, and sweet goodness. Most of these recipes are gluten free and refined sugar free. So go ahead and indulge . . . these treats are actually good for you!

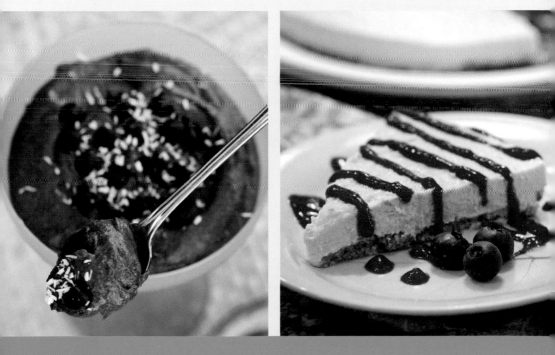

30 mini
bites

# Black Bean Brownie Bites

*Brownies are everyone's favorite, so I wanted to come up with a healthier version that was just as tasty. These bites are loaded with fiber yet still maintain the chocolaty goodness of a regular brownie. Your kids will love them, too!*

**To make date paste:** Pour two-thirds cup of hot water over one cup pitted dates and soak for about an hour. Put all of the ingredients into a blender and process until a smooth, thick paste is formed.

Preheat the oven to 350 degrees F. Grease mini muffin tins with coconut oil or coconut spray.

In a food processor with the S-blade, combine the black beans, banana, agave nectar, date paste, coconut oil, cacao powder, vanilla, cinnamon, and salt until well combined and smooth. Transfer the mixture to a large bowl.

Stir in the almond flour, baking powder, baking soda, and chocolate chips. Fill mini muffin tins about two-thirds full and bake 25 to 30 minutes or until a toothpick comes out clean. Remove from the oven and let them cool in the pan for 10 minutes, then transfer to a wire rack.

½ cup date paste (see recipe on left; allow 1 hour soaking time for dates)

Coconut oil or coconut spray for greasing pans

2 cups black beans (freshly cooked is best, but you can also use 1½ 15-ounce cans; drain the beans and rinse if using canned)

1 ripe banana

⅓ cup agave nectar

2 tablespoons melted coconut oil

½ cup raw cacao powder

1 tablespoon vanilla extract

1 tablespoon cinnamon

¼ teaspoon sea salt

¼ cup oat or almond flour

1 teaspoon baking powder

¼ teaspoon baking soda

½ cup grain-sweetened or vegan chocolate chips

Per Serving: Calories 80, Total Fat 3.5g, Saturated Fat 2g, Cholesterol 0mg, Sodium 50mg, Carbohydrate 13g, Fiber 3g, Protein 2g

195

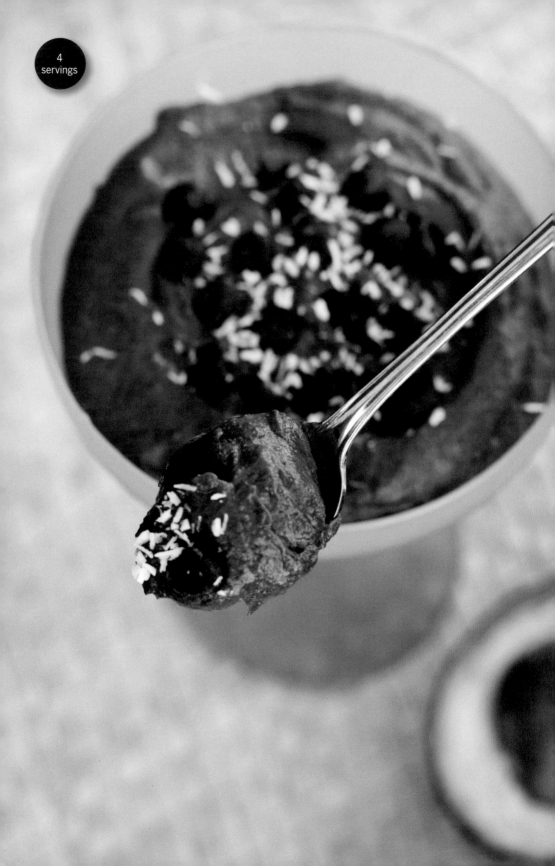

4
servings

# Choco Chocolate Chip Avo Pudding

*Yum! Chocolate pudding . . . my favorite!*
*This vegan and raw version is made with avocado and cashews.*
*When these two nutrient-rich ingredients are combined,*
*they make a smooth, velvety treat! It's best to use raw cacao powder,*
*as all the nutrients are intact and more available to the body.*

Drain the water from the cashews. Combine all of the ingredients except the chocolate chips in a blender and blend until smooth and creamy. Stir in the chocolate chips. Scoop into separate bowls and refrigerate for at least 2 hours to set.

1 cup cashews, soaked for 2 hours

2 ripe avocados

⅓ cup full-fat coconut milk

⅓ cup raw cacao powder

2 teaspoons vanilla extract

⅓ cup raw blue agave nectar or maple syrup

1 tablespoon arrowroot powder

¼ cup date paste (page 195)

1 tablespoon melted coconut oil

⅛ teaspoon fine sea salt

1 cup grain-sweetened or vegan chocolate chips

 **Karmic Health Tip:** *Did you know that soaking any kind of raw nut can help to cut the fat content by about half? So always allow time to soak your nuts before eating or cooking with them!*

## A Word About Alternative Sweeteners

There are many sweeteners available that are healthier for you than white sugar, but remember, they are still sugar and should be eaten minimally. Some of my favorites are raw blue agave nectar, grade B maple syrup, and brown rice syrup. These tend to be quite a bit lower on the glycemic index (GI) compared to white cane sugar. For instance, the GI for agave nectar is between 20–30, compared to 55 for honey and 68 for table sugar. There are also a lot of fancy names for sugar: evaporated cane juice, Sucanat, and raw sugar. Do your best to steer clear of these and use the alternatives I have listed in the "Alternative Sweet Stuff" section on page 20.

# Euphoria Nuggets

*These energy nuggets are great to make as a snack for your kids. Actually, your kids will love to help you make them! They are loaded with protein, healthy fats, natural sugars, and flavor. They are great for marathon runners or athletes who need to restore their glycogen levels on the go. Who needs a candy bar anyway?*

In a food processor, process the sunflower seeds and dates into a fine meal. Add the remaining ingredients and process until sticky and blended together. Refrigerate for 10 minutes to harden and then roll into one-inch balls.

1 cup shelled sunflower seeds

⅓ cup pitted dates

½ cup almonds

⅓ cup raw dark blue agave nectar

3–5 tablespoons raw cacao powder

Pinch of nutmeg and/or cinnamon

Pinch of sea salt

1 teaspoon vanilla extract

**Karmic Health Tip:** *Which do you use, raw cacao powder or processed cocoa powder? Raw cacao powder is the best choice as it's raw in nature and minimally processed, which keeps all of the natural alkalais and antioxidants of the cacao bean alive. Cocoa powder, which you can find in any grocery store, is usually overprocessed and stripped of its beneficial nutrients. If you can't find raw cacao powder near you, check out the Resources section on page 227 to order it online. A little goes a long way!*

Per Serving: Calories 90, Total Fat 5g, Saturated Fat 1g, Cholesterol 0mg, Sodium 0mg, Carbohydrate 9g, Fiber 2g, Protein 3g

 199

# Strawberry Crème Mousse with Pistachio Topping

4 servings

*I LOVE creamy, smooth, and fluffy mousse.
This version uses cashews and young Thai coconut meat,
which gives it a pleasing, smooth, mousselike texture. Topped with
crumbled pistachios, dates, and coconut, it's both crunchy and
velvety at the same time. Your taste buds will sing!*

Place all of the ingredients except the agave nectar in a food processor with the S-blade. Process until fully combined and then, with the motor running, pour in the agave nectar and blend until smooth. Pour into small cups and top with the Pistachio Topping (recipe follows). Refrigerate for about an hour so the mixture can gel. The topping should be chunky and not smooth, but still hold together.

2½ cups raw cashews or macadamia nuts, soaked for at least 2 hours

1 pint organic strawberries, hulled and cut in halves

¼ cup raw blue agave nectar or grade B maple syrup

Meat of 1 young Thai coconut (if not available, see tip on left)

Water from 1 young Thai coconut

1 teaspoon vanilla extract

1 tablespoon lemon juice

## Pistachio Topping

1 cup pistachios, raw or dry roasted without salt

¼ cup pitted dates

¼ cup raw, unsweetened shredded coconut

Dash of sea salt

2 tablespoons raw blue agave nectar

Per Serving: Calories 590, Total Fat 38g, Saturated Fat 7g, Cholesterol 0mg, Sodium 85mg, Carbohydrate 55g, Fiber 5g, Protein 17g
Pistachio Topping: Calories 260, Total Fat 17g, Saturated Fat 4.5g, Cholesterol 0mg, Sodium 0mg, Carbohydrate 25g, Fiber 5g, Protein 7g

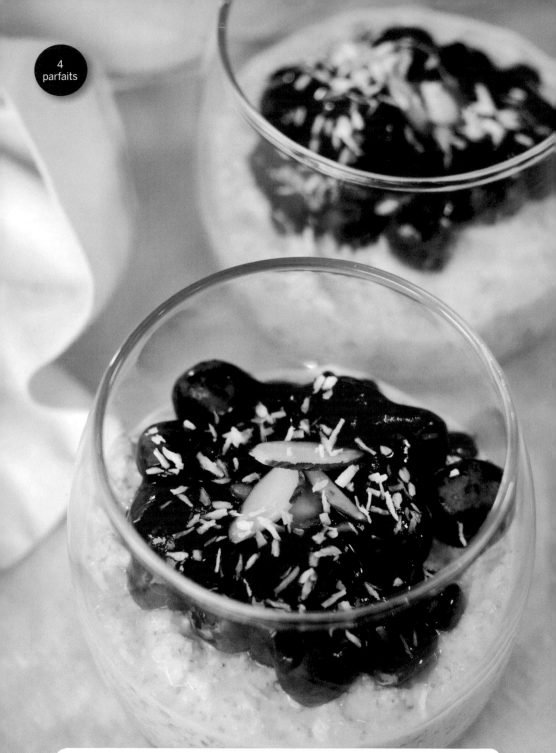

4
parfaits

**CHEF'S TIP**

If you don't like getting raspberry seeds stuck in your teeth, feel free to strain them through a fine sieve strainer for a more velvety sauce.

# Almond Berry Crème Parfaits

*I love parfaits, but when I stopped eating dairy, I didn't eat them for years.
I had to come up with another solution, so I created the Raw Almond
Frangipane Crème (see recipe below). Use any kind of berries
that are in season; and if it's winter, use apples!*

Place all of the ingredients in a blender or food processor and puree until thick and smooth. Add a touch more liquid if it's too thick.

### Raw Almond Frangipane Crème

1 cup almonds

1 cup coconut water

½ teaspoon almond extract

2 tablespoons maple syrup

Place all of the ingredients in a blender or food processor and puree until very smooth. You can strain the sauce if you don't like the seeds.

**To assemble the parfaits:** Layer the Raw Almond Frangipane Crème in a cup or wine glass; top the layer with the berries, and then top the berries with the raspberry sauce. Top with shredded coconut, granola, or nuts!

### Raspberry Sauce

1 10-ounce bag frozen raspberries, defrosted, or 2 pints fresh raspberries

¼ cup agave nectar

¼ cup water

¼ cup pitted soft dates

2 tablespoons lemon juice

2 cups fresh berries (assorted) or any kind of fresh fruit

Unsweetened, shredded coconut for topping

Per Serving (without shredded coconut): Calories 275, Total Fat 12g, Saturated Fat 1g, Cholesterol 0mg, Sodium 65mg, Carbohydrate 32g, Fiber 6g, Protein 7g

# Decadent Banana Carob Bread Pudding

*This recipe is a winner from a contest I ran
for my Karma Chow fans that challenged them to transform
their favorite decadent recipe into a healthier, veganized version.
Christy Griswold of Venice, California, created this
gluten-free beauty. Thank you, Christy, for bringing
bread pudding back into my life!*

Preheat the oven to 350 degrees F. Grease a 9 × 5-inch loaf pan. You can also make these in separate ramekin dishes for an elegant presentation, but you'll need to adjust cooking time to half.

Place the bread, bananas, and carob or chocolate chips in a large bowl. Set aside. In a blender or food processor, blend the milk, dates, and vanilla until smooth. Pour over the bread mixture and let it soak for 10 minutes. Pour it into the prepared pan. Line a roasting pan with a damp kitchen towel. Place the loaf pan on the towel inside the roasting pan, and place the roasting pan on the oven rack. Fill the roasting pan with hot water to reach halfway up the sides of the loaf pan. Bake for one hour, or until a knife inserted in the center comes out clean.

- 4 cups or 10 slices of cubed Ener-G Gluten Free Tapioca Bread or Ezekiel Sprouted Grain Cinnamon Raisin Bread
- 4 ripe bananas, mashed
- 10 ounces vegan carob chips or grain-sweetened chocolate chips
- 2 cups Cashew/Almond Milk (page 205)
- 12 dates, pitted and cut in half
- 1 tablespoon vanilla extract

Per Serving: Calories 460, Total Fat 19g, Saturated Fat 8g, Cholesterol 0mg, Sodium 40mg, Carbohydrate 78g, Fiber 9g, Protein 2g
Cashew/Almond Milk: Calories 130, Total Fat 6g, Saturated Fat 1.5g, Cholesterol 0mg, Sodium 170mg, Carbohydrate 15g, Fiber 3g, Protein 4g

Makes
3 cups

In a powerful blender or food processor, place the liquid from the coconut. Scrape the inside of the coconut meat into the blender using a spoon. Add the nuts and vanilla and blend into a smooth consistency. It should be thick like a cream. If the mixture appears to be too thick, add water or some additional coconut milk until the desired consistency is reached.

## Cashew/Almond Milk

Liquid and meat from
   1 young Thai coconut
   (should yield 16 ounces
   of liquid)

3 tablespoons almonds

3 tablespoons cashews

1 teaspoon vanilla extract

**CHEF'S TIP**

Short on time? Use store-bought almond or coconut milk for the recipe. Homemade raw nut milk is the best, but I understand we can all get busy, and we still want our dessert—and we want it now!

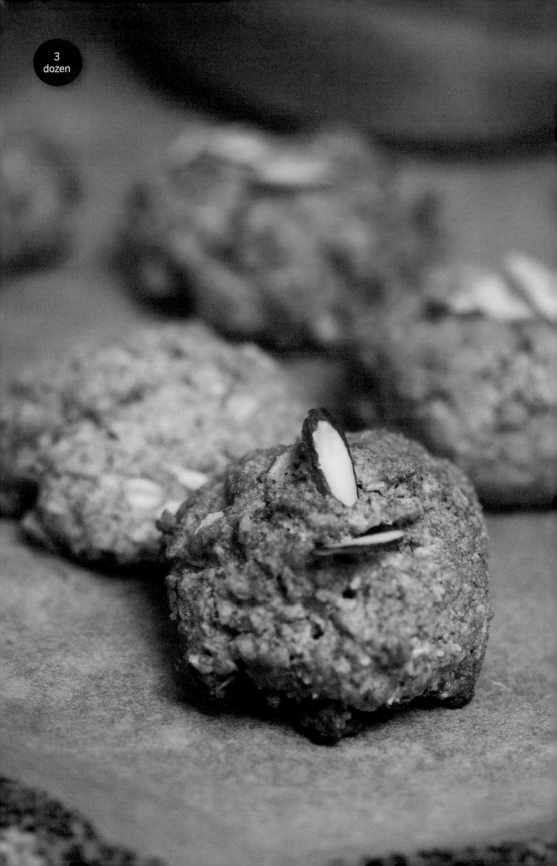

# Coconut Anise Almond Cookies

*These crunchy, nutty cookies are very simple to make once you grind the almonds and oats. I think you will enjoy the slight licorice flavor from the anise, but if you are not a fan of anise, just use almond extract for an extra nutty flavor! They are perfect at any holiday table.*

Preheat the oven to 350 degrees F. Combine all of the ingredients in a bowl and mix well. Drop by the teaspoonful onto cookie sheets lined with parchment paper. Place a couple of almond slices in the center of the cookie (optional). Bake for 10 to 12 minutes or until golden. Cool on a wire rack. These are great alone, but if you like chocolate, you can dip the cooled cookie in chocolate topping (recipe follows). These cookies are great for storing in the freezer and eating chilled!

1 cup spelt flour or oat flour (use gluten-free oat flour for gluten-free cookies)

¾ cup coarsely ground oats (use a blender or food processor to grind oats)

½ cup ground almonds or almond flour (use a food processor or coffee grinder to grind almonds)

¼ cup shredded, unsweetened coconut

½ cup agave nectar

1 teaspoon anise extract (use almond extract if anise is not available)

1 teaspoon cinnamon

½ cup melted coconut oil or avocado oil

2 tablespoons of unsweetened applesauce

1 teaspoon baking soda

½ teaspoon sea salt

Sliced almonds (optional, for garnish)

In a small saucepan over low heat, melt the chocolate chips with the milk and stir frequently until smooth.

## Chocolate Topping

1 cup grain-sweetened or vegan chocolate chips

2 tablespoons almond or coconut milk

Per Serving: Calories 70, Total Fat 4.5g, Saturated Fat 3g, Cholesterol 0mg, Sodium 70mg, Carbohydrate 7g, Fiber 1g, Protein 1g
Chocolate Topping: Calories 120, Total Fat 7g, Saturated Fat 5g, Cholesterol 0mg, Sodium 0mg, Carbohydrate 17g, Fiber 2g, Protein 0g

## Crumb Topping

2 cups rolled oats

1 cup oat or almond flour

½ cup toasted, sliced almonds

½ cup chopped walnuts

¼ teaspoon sea salt

½ cup agave nectar or brown rice syrup

⅓ cup grapeseed, melted coconut, or walnut oil

1 teaspoon almond extract

# Apple/Pear Crisp

*Apple crisp is one of America's favorite desserts.
I've added pears to this classic to give it a bit more flavor and
depth. Low-glycemic agave nectar, lower-sugar pears, and
Granny Smith apples make this dessert a healthier option.
This crisp is even more delectable when served with
Lavender Coconut Ice Cream on page 219.*

Preheat the oven to 350 degrees F. Peel, core, and slice the apples and pears in even one-quarter-inch to one-half-inch slices and place in a large bowl of water with lemon juice to prevent browning.

In a medium bowl, combine the agave nectar, almond extract, ginger, orange zest, and apple cider. Whisk in the arrowroot until dissolved.

Drain the apples and place them in a large casserole dish. Pour the agave mixture over the apples and pears, and set aside.

- 8–10 apples and pears total (Granny Smith, Fuji, and Bosc pears are a good mix)
- 2 tablespoons lemon juice
- ¼ cup agave nectar or maple syrup
- 1 teaspoon almond extract
- 2 teaspoons grated fresh ginger
- Zest of ½ an orange
- ½ cup pure apple cider or apple juice
- 1 tablespoon arrowroot powder

**To make the crumb topping:** In a food processor bowl using the S-blade, combine the oats, flour, almonds, walnuts, and salt. In another smaller bowl, whisk together the agave nectar, oil, and almond extract. Pour the agave mixture into the top of the processor and pulse until combined yet still chunky. Scrape out of processor bowl and sprinkle over the apples and pears in the casserole dish and spread out evenly. Cover with foil and bake for 35 minutes. Remove the foil and bake another 15 minutes until the topping is crisp and lightly brown. Remove from the oven and let it sit for 5 to 7 minutes to cool. Serve warm.

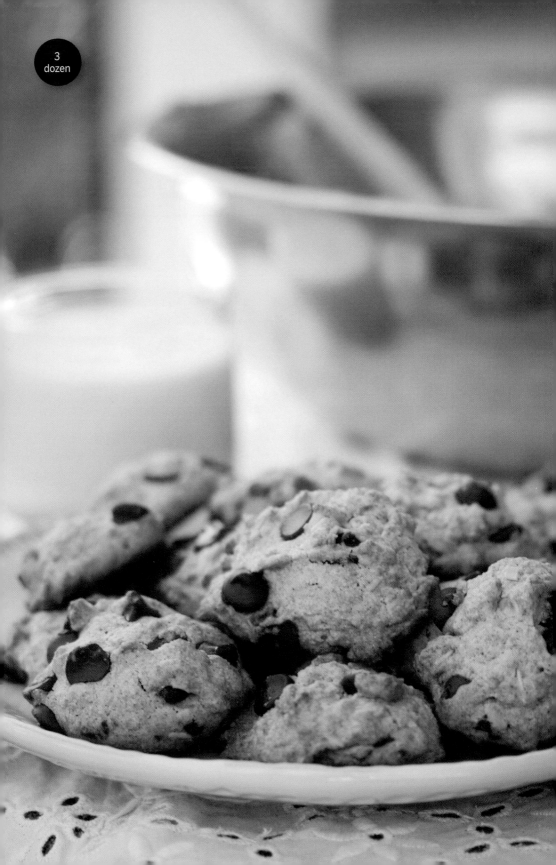

3
dozen

# Cardamom-Scented Chocolate Chippers

*So many people love chocolate chip cookies, and I think you'll*
*fall head over heels for this version. Cardamom is a warming spice*
*that is used a lot in Indian cooking, and it lends a sweet yet spicy flavor*
*to these cookies. These are a favorite among many of my clients,*
*including fitness expert and P90X™ creator Tony Horton.*

Preheat the oven to 350 degrees F. Combine the oat flour, oats, walnuts, salt, baking soda, cinnamon, cardamom, and chocolate chips in a bowl and whisk together to combine and break up any lumps. In another medium-size bowl, whisk together the agave nectar, coconut oil, milk, and vanilla until well combined. Pour the wet ingredients into the dry ingredients and stir together with a wooden spoon until well combined. Refrigerate for 10 minutes to firm the batter.

Place the batter by the tablespoonful on a baking sheet lined with parchment paper. Bake for 10 to 12 minutes or until golden brown. Remove and cool on a wire rack.

2 cups spelt or oat flour

¾ cup rolled oats

½ cup chopped walnuts (optional)

½ teaspoon sea salt

¾ teaspoon baking soda

⅛ teaspoon cinnamon

¼ teaspoon cardamom

1 cup grain-sweetened or vegan chocolate chips

⅔ cup agave nectar

⅔ cup melted coconut oil

2 tablespoons almond milk or coconut milk

1 teaspoon vanilla extract

Per Serving: Calories 120, Total Fat 7g, Saturated Fat 5g, Cholesterol 0mg, Sodium 60mg, Carbohydrate 13g, Fiber 1g, Protein 1g

# Divine Chocolate Truffles

*Truffles are my most favorite dessert on the planet.*
*These babies are actually good for you: they contain raw cacao,*
*which is packed with phytonutrients and enzymes.*
*These contain no refined sugars so they won't spike your blood sugar*
*levels like most store-bought truffles. Just one will do,*
*as they are so rich and satisfying.*

½ cup raw cashews

½ cup raw cacao butter, melted over very low heat

½ cup raw agave nectar (or ¼ cup agave plus ¼ cup maple syrup)

1 cup raw cacao powder (or ½ cup carob plus ½ cup cacao powder)

2 teaspoons vanilla extract (alcohol-free) or the seeds from ½ a vanilla bean

Pinch sea salt (preferably Himalayan Pink or Real Salt Sea Salt)

1 cup ground nuts, raw cacao nibs, cacao powder, or shredded coconut for rolling truffles (optional)

In a food processor fitted with the S-blade, process the cashews, melted cacao butter, and agave nectar until smooth. Add the cacao powder, vanilla extract, and salt, and process until well mixed and smooth. Scoop the mixture out into a large bowl and chill in the freezer for 10 to 20 minutes (the more chilled the mixture is, the easier it will be to roll into truffles). Once chilled, shape the mixture into walnut-size balls and then roll them in your choice of ground nuts, raw cacao nibs, cacao powder, or shredded coconut. Store in the refrigerator for up to two weeks or freeze for up to one month.

## CHEF'S TIP

 Be creative with this truffle recipe, according to your taste or the season: add goji berries, dried mulberries, mint extract, nuts—whatever you like to combine with chocolate.

Per Serving: Calories 130, Total Fat 9g, Saturated Fat 4g, Cholesterol 0mg, Sodium 10mg, Carbohydrate 10g, Fiber 3g, Protein 3g

# Peanut Butter Cookies

Preheat the oven to 350 degrees F. In a medium bowl, whisk together the flour, baking powder, baking soda, salt, and xanthan gum, and set aside. In another bowl, whisk together the applesauce, flaxseed eggs, vanilla, coconut oil, and the agave nectar until well combined. Add the peanut butter and stir to combine well. Using your hands, roll the dough into one-inch balls and place on a baking sheet lined with parchment, and then flatten with a fork. Bake for 10 to 12 minutes, until set but not hard. Cool on a wire rack.

2 cups Bob's Red Mill Gluten Free All Purpose Baking Flour

1 teaspoon baking powder

1 teaspoon baking soda

½ teaspoon salt

1 teaspoon xanthan gum

¼ cup plus 2 tablespoons applesauce

2 flaxseed eggs (page 26)

1 teaspoon vanilla extract

¼ cup melted coconut oil or avocado oil

½ cup agave nectar

½ cup peanut butter

16
squares

# Chocolaty Rice Krispy Thingies

*This recipe, inspired by chef Heather Crosby,
who founded the awesome vegan website Yum Universe,
is a modernized version of the Rice Krispies Treats we loved as kids,
which were unfortunately loaded with sugar. No marshmallows here,
but you will love these treats just as much as the originals!*

Grease the bottom of a 9 × 11-inch glass casserole dish using coconut oil. Using a food processor with the S-blade, process the almonds, sunflower seeds, oats, and sea salt until pulverized but still chunky. Pour into a large bowl along with 1 cup of the vegan chocolate chips and the brown rice crispy cereal.

Meanwhile, in a small saucepan over low heat, combine the cashew butter, rice syrup, coconut oil, and vanilla extract, stirring constantly until the cashew butter is melted and combined with the rice syrup. Pour the cashew butter mixture over the dry ingredients and stir well to coat evenly. Fold into the greased casserole dish.

1 cup raw almonds

⅔ cup raw sunflower seeds

⅓ cup rolled oats

½ teaspoon sea salt

1 bag (16 ounces) of vegan or grain-sweetened chocolate chips

2 cups brown rice crispy cereal

¼ cup cashew butter or peanut butter

¾ cup organic brown rice syrup

1 tablespoon melted coconut oil

1 teaspoon vanilla extract

Using a double boiler, melt the remaining chocolate chips and stir until smooth. (If you don't have a double boiler, melt the chips directly in a saucepan over very low heat while constantly stirring.) Spread the melted chocolate over the rice mixture evenly and refrigerate for at least 2 hours to set. Once set, cut into small squares. Keep refrigerated in a tightly covered glass storage container.

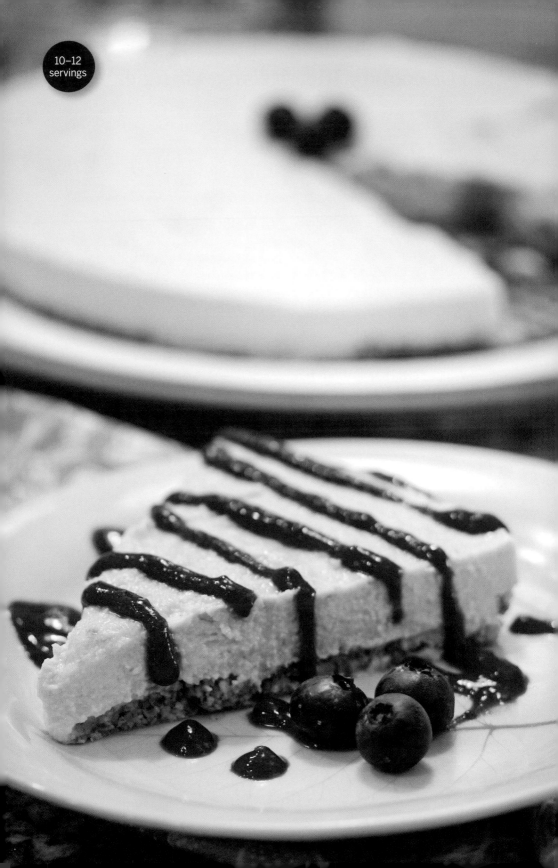

# Luscious Limey "Cheese"cake

*I loved cheesecake as a kid, but I knew how unhealthy it was for me.
This dairy-free version is creamy, citrusy, and delightful, a counterpart
to the original without all the unhealthy sugar and fat!
The filling is made with cashews, which provide a lot of
nutrients and healthy fats. It's delicious topped with
my simple Raspberry Sauce (page 203).*

**Making the crust:** In a food processor, pulse the nuts, agave nectar, coconut, and sea salt together until sticky. Press into a 9-inch springform pan.

**Making the filling:** In a blender, blend all of the filling ingredients together until smooth and creamy. If the mixture is too thick, add a bit more coconut water. Pour into the crust and freeze for 1 to 2 hours until firm. Open the springform pan, remove the rim, and place the cake on a plate. Slice while frozen and defrost for about a half hour to soften up before serving, depending on how frozen the cheesecake is.

## Crust

2 cups nuts (walnuts, macadamias, or pecans)

¼ cup agave nectar

½ cup shredded, unsweetened coconut

¼ teaspoon sea salt

## Filling

3 cups cashews, soaked for 4 hours

1 cup pitted and chopped dates, soaked for 2 hours

6 tablespoons melted coconut oil

½ cup lime juice

½ cup agave nectar

4 tablespoons coconut water

Seeds from one vanilla bean, or 2 teaspoons vanilla extract

**Karmic Health Tip:** *Did you know that a handful of raw cashews a day can help keep depression away? The latest studies are showing this to be true!*

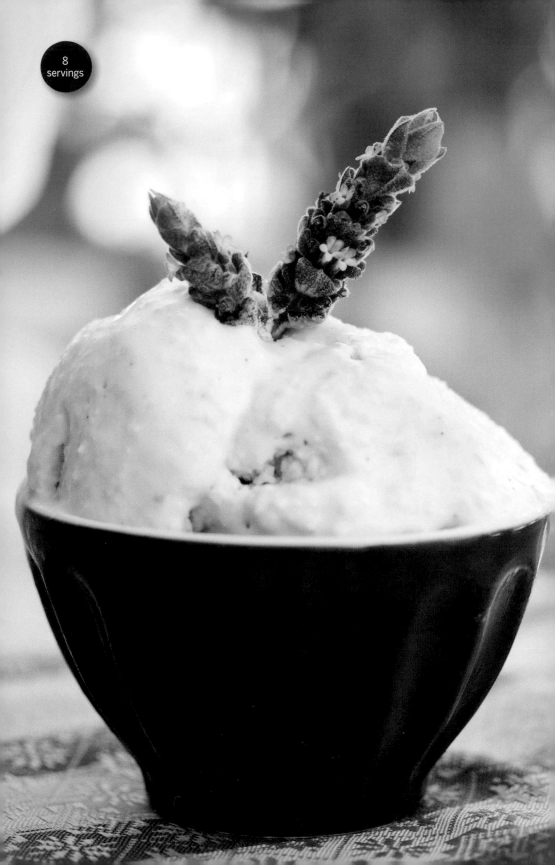

# Lavender Coconut Ice Cream

*Ice cream is one dessert that I was sad to give up when I became vegan. This nut milk—based vegan ice cream is simple to make, and its creamy consistency is just like what you would buy in the grocery store, but it's healthier for you! Adding dried lavender gives it an exotic, fresh flavor.*

Blend all of the ingredients together in a high-speed blender and blend until smooth and creamy. Pour into frozen ice-cream maker bowl and follow the manufacturer's instructions.

Allow to thaw 10 to 15 minutes before serving.

1 cup cashews, soaked for 30 minutes

2 cups full-fat coconut milk

⅓ cup agave nectar or maple syrup

1 tablespoon ground, dried lavender

Seeds from 1 vanilla bean or 1 tablespoon vanilla extract

¼ cup shredded, unsweetened coconut

¼ teaspoon sea salt

¼ cup melted coconut oil

 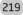

**About 2 cups**

# Coconut Whipped Cream

*This whipped cream is dairy free, decadent, and delicious.*
*Spoon it onto my Luscious Limey "Cheese"cake, over ice cream, or*
*on pie. Its smooth, creamy texture is just like the real thing.*
*You can add cinnamon, cardamom, or any other*
*spice you like for different variations.*

1 15-ounce can full-fat coconut
milk, stored in the fridge for
3 hours

1 teaspoon vanilla extract

1 tablespoon agave nectar
(more if you like it sweeter)

Open the coconut milk and spoon out the top layer of the thickened coconut cream. Leave the remaining milky liquid in the can and use it for smoothies or for other recipes. Place the coconut cream in a bowl and whip with electric beaters starting on low and moving to high until creamy. Move beaters up and down to infuse with lots of air as mixing. Add in the vanilla and agave nectar and stir to combine. This keeps in the refrigerator for three days in a container with a tight-fitting lid.

Per Serving: Calories 60, Total Fat 6g, Saturated Fat 5g, Cholesterol 0mg, Sodium 0mg, Carbohydrate 2g, Fiber 0g, Protein 1g

# Vanilla Scented Balsamic Figs

*I love fresh figs, and these are awesome served on top of
ice cream or vegan yogurt. You can even layer them in my Rise and
Shine Granola Parfaits on page 39 or spread them on whole grain
toast with almond butter. If you cannot find fresh figs or
they are out of season, use dried mission figs.*

Combine all of the ingredients in a saucepan and bring to a boil. Lower the heat and simmer until the sauce starts to become thick and syrupy, about 10 to 15 minutes.

- 1 pint fresh figs, stems removed and quartered (or use a half pint of dried figs)
- ¼ cup balsamic vinegar
- ¼ cup apple juice or water
- 3 tablespoons maple syrup
- 1 teaspoon vanilla extract or seeds from 1 vanilla bean

# Baked Coconut Ginger Millet Pudding

*I love rice pudding, and this version is even better because it contains millet, which is high in minerals and protein and is also known to boost serotonin, which calms and soothes us. You can even eat this for breakfast with some fresh fruit on top, as it's healthy enough!*

2 cups almond milk

1 cup coconut milk

¾ cup millet

1 cup shredded, unsweetened coconut

2 tablespoons fresh grated ginger

1 teaspoon cinnamon

¼ cup dried cherries or cranberries

¼ cup maple syrup

1 teaspoon sea salt

1 teaspoon vanilla extract

1 tablespoon coconut oil plus more for greasing dish

Preheat the oven to 350 degrees F. Grease a casserole dish with coconut oil or cooking spray. In a large saucepan, heat both milks to scalding but not boiling. Add the remaining ingredients to the saucepan and stir together until combined. Pour the mixture into the casserole dish and cook in the oven for 90 minutes until the millet is soft. If the pudding seems dry, add a bit more coconut milk. Serve with fresh fruit or jam on top.

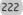 Per Serving: Calories 470, Total Fat 31g, Saturated Fat 25g, Cholesterol 0mg, Sodium 680mg, Carbohydrate 47g, Fiber 6g, Protein 6g

# Baking Substitutions 101

*B*elow are some substitutions you can use when baking in case you are at a loss making sense of all the fancy flours, sweeteners, and thickeners. Keep in mind that these conversions will vary from recipe to recipe and from one renowned chef to another. Remember, baking is a science, and one batch of cookies can come out different than the next batch, even if you follow the recipe to a T! Even simple techniques, such as the way you stir or fold in the ingredients, can affect the final product.

**To substitute for 1 cup of white flour:**

| | |
|---|---|
| 1⅜ cups barley flour | ⅞ cup rice flour |
| 1 cup buckwheat flour | 1 cup rye meal |
| 1 cup corn flour | 1 cup oat flour |
| ⅞ cup cornmeal | 1 cup whole wheat flour |
| ⅜ cup potato flour | |

Experiment with mixing different flours together to create more flavor and texture. *Note:* Always use a double portion of baking powder when using dark flour like buckwheat or rye.

## To substitute for 1 cup of whole wheat flour:

⅞ cup amaranth

1 cup buckwheat flour

¾ cup corn flour

1 cup cornmeal

⅞ cup garbanzo bean flour (chickpea)

¾ cup millet flour

¾ cup oat flour

⅝ cup potato flour

¾ cup potato starch

⅞ cup rice flour
  (white or brown)

¾ cup soy flour

1 cup spelt flour

## Cornstarch substitution:

Use arrowroot, kuzu, or corn flour. Corn flour thickens sauces better than cornstarch and may be used in the same proportions as white flour. It also combines well with other flours when making muffins.

## To substitute 1 cup of white sugar:

¾ cup maple syrup (when using maple syrup, reduce the liquid in the recipe by 3 tablespoons)

¾ cup plus 1 tablespoon honey (when using honey, reduce the liquid in the recipe by 2 tablespoons)

¾ cup agave nectar (when using agave, reduce the liquid in the recipe by 3 tablespoons)

1⅓ cups molasses (when using molasses, reduce the liquid in the recipe by 5 tablespoons and add ½ teaspoon baking soda for each cup of molasses used. Do not replace more than half the sugar in a recipe with molasses.)

1 cup palm or coconut sugar

1½ cups brown rice syrup (when using brown rice syrup, reduce the liquid in the recipe by 3 tablespoons)

1 cup date sugar

1½ cups barley malt syrup (when using barley malt syrup, reduce the liquid in the recipe by 2 tablespoons)

## What Can I Use Instead of Eggs When I Bake?

I get this question all the time, and there are a lot of alternatives out there for baking without eggs. Here are some suggestions that I find work well. Keep in mind that the desserts in this book are healthier, so they won't always have the same exact fluffy texture as what you may be used to, but I promise they will have the flavor you crave!

**To substitute for 1 egg when baking:**

1 tablespoon ground flaxseed or chia seeds whipped in a blender with 3 tablespoons of water (let it sit until it gels)

¼ cup applesauce, canned pumpkin or squash, or pureed prunes (when using these, add an extra ½ teaspoon baking powder to make the recipe less dense)

Ener-G Egg Replacer (follow the instructions on the box)

½ ripe banana, mashed

2 tablespoons cornstarch beaten with 2 tablespoons of water

# Resources
# and Recommendations

*I realize that some of you* may live in areas where it's hard to find all the ingredients listed in this cookbook, so I am providing you with some of my favorite resources below. I like to buy a lot of my dried ingredients online as it saves money. This also helps me to keep my kitchen stocked and ready to go so I can whip up a healthy meal in a pinch. I have also included great places to buy knives and other kitchen ware!

**Amazon.com**
www.amazon.com
Groceries, supplements, appliances

**Bob's Red Mill**
www.bobsredmill.com
Dried foods, grains, beans, nuts

**Essential Living Foods**
http://www.essentiallivingfoods.com/
Raw nuts, maca, cacao, nuts

**Frontier Co-op**

www.frontierco-op/com

Bulk organic herbs, dried foods, spices, teas, and essential oils

**Navitas Naturals**

www.navitasnaturals.com

Maca, goji berries, raw cacao

**Vegan Essentials**

www.veganessentials.com

Clothing, specialty vegan food, raw vegan cheeses

**Veganstore**

www.veganstore.com

Clothing, shoes, food, supplements

Vitacost

www.vitacost.com

Organic and gluten-free flours, crackers, supplements, and so on

## Meal Delivery
### (Vegan and Plant-Based Options Nationwide)

**Fresh and Lean**

www.freshandlean.com

**Thrive Foods Direct**

www.thrivefoodsdirect.com

**TH KITCHEN**

www.tonyhortonkitchen.com

# Kitchen Gear

*Knives, appliances, cutting boards, etc. Here are some of my favorite sites that offer high quality kitchen gear.*

**Wayfair.com**—Everything you can imagine for your kitchen all on one site!

**Sur La Table**—High quality, beautiful, and somewhat pricey selection of every kitchen utensil you can imagine.

**Bed, Bath & Beyond**—Great for appliances, juicers, cutting boards, glass jars, and storage.

**Chef's Catalog.com**—An awesome array of chef-quality items.

## Favorite Blogs and Healthy Recipe Sites

Choosing Raw (http://www.choosingraw.com/)

The Blissful Chef (http://theblissfulchef.com/)

Gluten Free Goddess (http://glutenfreegoddess.blogspot.com/)

Healthy Voyager (http://healthyvoyager.com/2.0/)

Oh She Glows (http://ohsheglows.com/)

Spunky Coconut (http://www.thespunkycoconut.com/)

Vegweb (http://vegweb.com/)

Yum Universe (http://www.yumuniverse.com/)

## Apps for iPhone and Smart Phones

Eden Recipes • How to Cook Everything Vegetarian

Produce Guide • Vegetarian Cookbook • VegOut • Whole Foods

# Books and Films

Brazier, Brendan. 2008. *Thrive: The Vegan Nutrition Guide to Optimal Performance in Sports and Life*. Cambridge, MA: Da Capo Lifelong Books.

———. 2011. *Thrive Foods: 200 Plant-Based Recipes for Peak Health*. Cambridge, MA: Da Capo Lifelong Books.

Campbell II, Thomas M., and T. Colin Campbell. 2006. *The China Study: The Most Comprehensive Study of Nutrition Ever Conducted and the Startling Implications for Diet, Weight Loss, and Long-Term Health*. Dallas, TX: BenBella Books.

*Fat, Sick & Nearly Dead*. 2010. Documentary. Written and directed by Joe Cross and Kurt Engfehr. Story by Joe Cross and Robert Mac.

*Food, Inc.* 2008. Documentary. Directed by Robert Kenner.

*Forks over Knives*. 2011. Documentary. Written and directed by Lee Fulkerson.

*Hungry For Change*, DVD. Dr. Alejandro Junger, 2012.

Fuhrman, Joel. 2001. *Eat to Live: The Amazing Nutrient-Rich Program for Fast and Sustained Weight Loss*. Rev. ed. New York: Little, Brown, and Company.

Kessler, David. 2010. *The End of Overeating: Taking Control of the Insatiable American Appetite*. Emmaus, PA: Rodale.

Norris, Jack, and Virginia Messina. 2011. *Vegan for Life: Everything You Need to Know to Be Healthy and Fit on a Plant-Based Diet*. Cambridge, MA: Da Capo Lifelong Books.

Pollan, Michael. 2007. *Omnivore's Dilemma: A Natural History of Four Meals*. New York: Penguin.

Robbins, John. 1998. *Diet for a New America*. Novato, CA: H. J. Kramer.

Wolcott, William Linz, and Trish Fahey. 2002. *The Metabolic Typing Diet: Customize Your Diet to Your Own Unique Body Chemistry*. New York: Three Rivers Press.

# Acknowledgments

*T*o everyone who made this book possible, I am beyond grateful. First and foremost, I want to thank Tony Horton for his continued support, friendship, and inspiration. Without him this book would've not come to be. Also, thank you to Allison Janse for finding me, working with me, and always supporting my vision—and special thanks to HCI and everyone there who worked so hard to make this book happen.

I would like to thank my dear friend Jill for all her support and love through the process, especially for whisking me off to Santa Barbara to put the finishing touches on the book and for her awesome eating capabilities during the photo shoot! I am so grateful to my family for their support and belief in me, especially my mom, who has always allowed me to follow my heart. Thank you to my soul sister, Karen, for always being my biggest cheerleader. I would also like to thank my amazing classmates at the University of Santa Monica for unconditionally loving me and prizing me. Erinn, thank you for the diligent hours you spent editing my recipes and getting cozy with my garbage disposal. To all my recipe testers and committed Karma Chow followers who lovingly offered their feedback on what tasted good and what didn't, thank you. To Lizanne, Carrie, and Kyle for being diligent dishwashers and kitchen supporters. Others I would like to extend my thanks to include Heather Hayward for helping me to realize my passion of cooking for others, my Women's Power Group for their inspiration and unending support of my vision to create this cookbook, and Katina Stallworth at Whole Foods Market in West Los Angeles for collaborating with me to lead monthly cooking classes so that I can bring delicious, plant-based food to the masses. Thank you to all the Beachbody and Tony Horton fans who crave healthy food and begged for a cookbook from me, to the beautiful and talented chef Agi Harkins of One More Bite for contributing three awesome recipes to my repertoire, and to the crew at Food & Flow, especially Hari Bhajan, for helping to bring Karma Chow cooking to the Internet. I am especially grateful to my Gram for teaching me how to bake at such a young age and to my dad, may he rest in peace, for his Italian expertise in the kitchen. My four-legged canine lovebug, Pumpkin, has provided unconditional love and support through it all. And an extra special thanks to Kelsey Skiver of Kelsey Marie Photo for making my creations come alive with her beautiful photos and talented photography. And finally, a huge thank-you to all the other amazing vegan chefs and bloggers out there who continue to inspire me daily.

# About the Author

*Raised in New Jersey,* on the typical American SAD diet, Melissa Costello became passionate about healthy food at a young age. Her battle with multiple childhood illnesses led her to learn more about how the food we put in our bodies has a direct correlation to how healthy we are.

After Melissa gave up eating red meat at the age of nineteen, her passion for cooking led her to experiment with healthier, plant-based foods. Finding ways to make these foods taste good was the beginning of her life-long journey into culinary nutrition. She eventually completed a Nutrition Certification at NHI in San Diego, as Melissa knew she wanted to bring this passion to others and teach them about the benefits of healthy eating.

As a self-taught chef who loved to throw dinner parties, many of Melissa's friends told her she needed to cook for a living. Melissa started Karma Chow, her successful personal chef and coaching business in 2008. Her very first client was Tony Horton, the creator of the wildly popular home workout system, P90X. Melissa worked with Tony to help fuel his body with healthy, delicious foods so that he could thrive in his workouts and keep his energy sustained throughout his busy schedule.

Melissa continues to cook, teach, and lecture throughout the United States. She is continually finding innovative ways to bring her knowledge of healthy eating to the world. Her popular Vital Life 30-Day food-based cleanse has changed the lives of thousands across the country. Learn more at: www.karmachow.com.

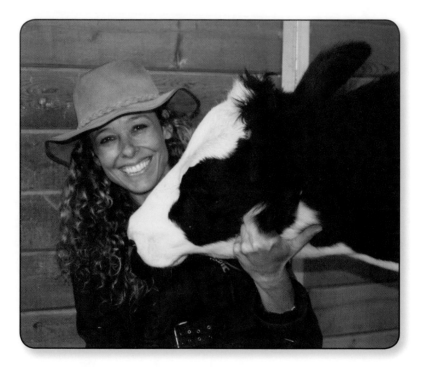

# Index

**A**

almonds
  berry crème parfait, 203
  breakfast bowl, 25
  coconut anise cookies, 207
  granola, 33
  roasted, 83
aluminum cookware, 10–11
Anaheim chilies
  ranchero sauce, 89
agave, 17, 21, 198
apple
  cherry chutney, 173
  crisp, 209
artichoke heart
  bruschetta, 71
  spinach dip, 81
  white bean dip, 73
asthma, 4
avocado
  gazpacho, 99
  mayo, 90


**B**

bakeware, 10–11
baking, 19–20, 28
  substitutions, 223–224
balsamic vinegar
  maple salad dressing, 121
banana
  bread pudding, 204

chocolate chip muffins, 29
chia pancakes, 43
smoothie, 44
beans
  black bean dip, 75
  black bean tropical soup, 96
  buying in bulk, 15
  cooking, 15
  shepherd's pie, 143
  white bean dip, 73
  white bean soup, 109
bell pepper
  breakfast scramble, 31
  quinoa stuffed, 161
benefits of plant-based diet, 2
black bean
  brownies, 195
  dip, 75
  tropical soup, 96
blender, 13
blueberries
  breakfast parfait, 39
  smoothie, 44
bowls, mixing and prep, 12
Bragg's amino acids, 17
bread, 18
  zucchini, 56
bread pudding
  banana, 204
breakfast scramble, 31
brownies
  black beans, 195

bruschetta
    artichoke heart, 71
Brussels sprouts
    maple miso, 177
    salad, 115
buckwheat
    corn cakes, 37
burritos
    rice, 155


C

cabbage
    red Dijon slaw, 139
    sweet and sour, 172
    Thai slaw, 127
Caesar salad, 134
calorie counting, 7
candy, 3
carrot
    cauliflower soup, 111
cashew
    chipotle cheese sauce, 85
    ice cream, 219
    milk, 41
    soba noodle stir-fry, 141
cast-iron cookware, 11
cauliflower
    carrot soup, 111
    cilantro smash, 186
    cumin roasted, 191
celery
    cream of celery soup, 103
chemicals in food, 9
cherry
    apple chutney, 173
    chocolate smoothie, 47
    granola, 33
    pecan quinoa muffins, 53
chia seeds
    banana pancakes, 43
chicken, 5
chickpeas
    burgers, 163
    fillets, 149
    herb salad, 123
    salad, 157
chili, tempeh, 112

chili peppers (see also individual varieties)
    ranchero sauce, 89
chipotle
    cashew sauce, 85
    mayo, 163
    salad dressing, 117
chips, 3
chocolate
    banana muffins, 29
    cherry smoothie, 47
    chip cookies, 211
    hot chocolate, 45
    pudding, 197
    Rice Krispy treats, 215
    truffles, 212
cholesterol, 3
cleansing, 7
coconut
    anise almond cookies, 207
    banana pancakes, 43
    chai, 51
    ginger millet pudding, 222
    ice cream, 219
    milk, 50
    peanut sauce, 84
    yam soup, 95
    whipped cream, 220
    whole, 200
coconut creamer, 19
coconut flakes
    breakfast bowl, 25
coconut palm sugar, 21
coffee grinder, 12
cookware, 10–11
corn
    buckwheat cakes, 37
    chowder, 101
curry
    greens, 187
    tempeh salad, 158
    veggie soup, 106
cutting boards, 10


D

deglazing, 60
dieting, 6
digestive health, 4
dip

artichoke and white bean, 73
artichoke spinach, 81
black bean, 75
edamame, 65
green Earth dip, 69
hummus, 67

**E**

Earth Balance spread, 18
eating disorders, 4
edamame, 17
    dip, 65
egg replacements, 18
eggs, 5
    substitutions, 225
enchilada
    casserole, 164

**F**

fajita, 153
fat, dietary, 4
figs
    balsamic vanilla, 221
flaxseed eggs, 26
flours, 20
food processor, 13

**G**

gazpacho
    avocado, 99
ginger
    coconut pudding, 222
    tea, 45
gluten, 2, 5
glycemic index, 20, 198
greens, baby
    salad, 133
granola
    cherry almond, 33
    parfait, 39
grater, 11–12
green beans
    cranberry balsamic, 171
greens (*see also* kale *and* spinach)
    curried, 187

**H**

herbs, stocking, 16
hummus
    garnet yam, 67
Horton, Tony, 6
hot dogs, 3

**I**

illness, 4
inflammation, 3

**J**

jars, glass, 13

**K**

kale
    chips, 86
    green smoothie, 49
    salad with chipotle dressing, 117
    slaw, 129
    tahini, 181
    white bean soup, 109
ketchup, 17
kidney beans
    shepherd's pie, 143
kiwi
    smoothie, 44
knives, buying, 9–10
kombu, 15

**L**

lakanto, 21
lemon
    dill aioli dipping sauce, 148
lentil
    soup, 93
lettuce
    tempeh wrap, 59
lime
    vinaigrette, 125

**M**

macaroni and cheese, 147
Magic Bullet, 13

maple syrup, 21, 198
"meat" balls, 137
microplanes, 11–12
migraines, 4
milk, dairy free, 17
miso, 17–18
molasses, blackstrap, 20
mortar and pestle, 12
muffins
    apricot tea, 27
    cherry pecan 53
mushrooms
    breakfast scramble, 31
    fajitas, 153
    gravy, 88
    quinoa pilaf, 169
    poppers, 61
mustard, 18

**N**

nonstick cookware, 10–11
nori
    veggie roll-up, 63
nut butter, 18
nuts
    cheesecake, 217
    toasted, 138

**O**

oats
    cinnamon cereal, 40
    granola, 33
olives
    tapenade, 78

**P**

P90X, 6
pad thai, 144
pain, 3
pantry, stocking with basics, 14
pasta, gluten free, 18
    "meat" balls, 137
    pesto, tomato and zucchini, 159
peanut butter
    cookies, 213

peanuts
    sauce, 84
pears
    crisp, 209
peas
    pesto, 175
    yellow split pea soup, 102
pecan
    cherry quinoa muffins, 53
    roasted, 83
peeler, 11
pesto
    pasta, 159
    soba noodle, 175
pistachios
    roasted, 83
planning menus, 3, 21–22
popcorn, 79
Pop-Tarts, 3
potatoes
    dill salad, 122
    mashed topping, 142
potatoes, red
    herb roasted, 185
pressure cooker, 13, 15
processed food, 2–4
pudding
    chocolate, 197
pumpkin
    pie waffles, 55
pumpkin seed
    salad dressing, 129

**Q**

quinoa
    breakfast bowl, 25
    cherry pecan muffins, 53
    mushroom pilaf, 169
    strawberry salad, 125
    stuffed peppers, 161
    tabbouleh, 119

**R**

raisins
    breakfast bowl, 25
raspberries
    almond crème parfaits, 203
    breakfast parfait, 39

rice
    burrito, 155
    syrup, 198
    veggie loaf, 150
    wild rice salad, 121
rice cooker, 13
rice noodles
    pad Thai, 144
rice syrup, 21
romaine lettuce
    Caesar salad, 134
    green smoothie, 49

**S**

salad spinner, 12
salt, sea, 19
santoku knives, 10
shepherd's pie, 143
sleep, 2
soba noodles
    cashew stir-fry, 141
    pesto, 175
soy, 17
spatula, 12
spelt, 120
spices, stocking, 16
spinach
    artichoke dip, 81
    baked ziti, 154
    garlic, 189
    green smoothie, 49
    salad, 131
squash, butternut
    soup, 104–105
squash, spaghetti
    Italiano, 179
stevia, 21
strainer, 11
strawberries
    breakfast parfait, 39
    mousse, 201
    quinoa salad, 125
    smoothie, 44
sugar, 2–5, 198
sunflower seed
    dessert nuggets, 199
    pate, 77

sushi
    rolling, 62
    veggie seed roll-ups, 63
sweet potatoes
    chili batons, 178

**T**

tabbouleh, quinoa, 119
tacos
    tempeh, 139
tahini
    dressing, 131
    kale, 181
tamari, 17, 19
tapenade
    olives, 78
tea
    coconut chai, 51
    ginger, 45
tempeh, 17, 19
    chili, 112
    curry salad, 158
    enchiladarole, 164
    lettuce wrap, 59
    sausage patties, 35
    stew, 107
    tacos, 139
tomatoes
    Greek burgers, 145
    marinara, 87
    pasta, 159
tofu, 17
tortilla, 18
traditional eating habits, 8–9
truffles, dessert, 212

**V**

Vegenaise, 19
vegetable loaf, 150
vegetable soup, 97

**W**

waffles
    pumpkin pie, 55
walnuts
    pear and pomegranate dressing, 133
    roasted, 83

weight loss, 1
white beans
    dip, 73
    soup, 109
    tomato burgers, 145
    zucchini salad, 132
wooden spoons, 12
Worcestershire sauce, 19, 136
wrap
    tempeh lettuce, 59


## X

xanthan gum, 19


## Y

yam
    breakfast scramble, 31
    coconut soup, 95
    hummus, 67
    mashed with coconut, 183
yeast flakes, 18
    popcorn, 79


## Z

ziti, baked, 154
zucchini
    bread, 56
    breakfast scramble, 31
    pasta, 159
    white bean salad, 132